Legally Safe Mental Health Practice:
Psycholegal Questions and Answers

Legally Safe Mental Health Practice:

Psycholegal Questions and Answers

ROBERT HENLEY WOODY, PH.D., SC.D., J.D.

PSYCHOSOCIAL PRESS
MADISON, CONNECTICUT

Library of Congress Cataloging-in-Publication Data

Woody, Robert Henley.
    Legally safe mental health practice : psycholegal questions and answers / Robert Henley Woody.
       p.   cm.
    Includes bibliographical references.
    ISBN 1-887841-04-0
    1. Mental health personnel—Malpractice. 2. Mental health personnel—Professional ethics.   I. Title.
RC440.8.W6595 1997
616.89'0068—dc20
                                           96-30831
                                            CIP

Contents

Dedication

This book is dedicated to the mental health practitioners to whom I have provided legal services. While I trust that they have benefited from my counsel, I readily acknowledge that I have learned a great deal from their sharing of their personal and professional lives with me.

I also dedicate this book to my family—Jane, Jennifer, Robert III, and Matthew—for their continued love and support.

A Cautionary Note

This book is intended to provide information for educational purposes only. It is sold with the understanding that the publisher and author are not engaged in rendering legal or other professional services herein, and do not warrant the applicability for any situation in which the reader may be engaged. Specifically, the answers to the questions are for exemplary and/or educational purposes, and their suitability for particular usage will be contingent upon unique facts and the jurisdiction relevant to the reader. If legal advice or other expert assistance is required, the services of a competent professional, with knowledge of all laws pertaining to the reader, should be obtained.

Foreword

Mental health practitioners are on the threshold of unprecedented conditions for professional services. As the twenty-first century approaches, American society has problems that create challenges to mental health care providers that will be difficult to meet. Society recognizes that mental health professionals have valuable expertise, which could provide remedies. Nonetheless, society imposes economic conditions, especially under the health care reform movement, that restrict the availability and quality of mental health services. In many ways, it seems that, almost inexplicably, there has been a diminution of priority for supporting mental health, notwithstanding the profound cries for help emanating from all sectors of society.

The health care reform movement demands reduced costs for services, more accountability by providers, and alternative (lesser trained and less expensive) providers. All three of these criteria are pressing mental health professionals to lower the standard of care. The marketplace is now rife with practitioners with so few qualifications that a short time ago they would have been blocked from providing services to the public. Fees for services have dropped and continue to drop precipitously. Even highly trained practitioners find themselves tempted to perform in a second-rate fashion.

To exacerbate the situation, today's mental health practitioner is under intense scrutiny for possible legal action, by clients, third-party payment sources (e.g., insurance carriers, managed health care systems), and government regulators. There is a proliferation of legal complaints to state licensing boards and consumer protection agencies, as well as the malpractice courts.

At this point in time, the mental health practitioner must take drastic steps to survive. That is, the financial and legal considerations do not accommodate a "business as usual" attitude. There must be a renovation of operations and practices directed at meeting the threats and challenges. This book is directed at this objective.

In 1960, I started my professional career as a psychologist. Becoming a professor in 1964, I soon moved into private practice as well. By the early 1970s, I was immersed in attempting to sort out the best ways to deliver services to the entire community. Soon, however, the community mental health movement, birthed in the Great Society years, met its demise. By the 1980s, it was clear that entrepreneurship was the hallmark of successful mental health practice. By then, I was an attorney, aware that "times they are a-changin' " for mental health practitioners.

Since 1981, my law practice has been devoted primarily to protecting mental health practitioners from complaints (ethical, regulatory or licensing, and malpractice) and providing these practitioners with information from business law. Moving from psychology to law has been an enriching experience for me—I have gained more understanding of the therapist-client relationship from the vantage point of being an attorney than I ever recognized during my years as a psychologist. My clients—psychologists, social workers, marriage and family therapists, professional counselors, and psychiatrists—have shared their therapeutic experiences with me, and together we have sought to find enhanced strategies for producing practice success and avoiding legal problems.

This book contains a collection of actual questions that have been posed to me by my clients. Some of the questions may seem unbelievable, but except for paraphrasing for clarity or to protect anonymity, the questions and scenarios are real. Rereading the final manuscript led to my realizing that, surprisingly, virtually every question has been asked by multiple sources, with only slight variations.

Regrettably, some of the situations reflect bad judgment, nefarious motives, pathological conditions, and intentional violations of ethics and the law by the mental health practitioner. After my years as a psychologist believing in the unrestricted goodness of the person, I now know that I was quite naive. I must quickly add that this naivete extended to unconditional positive regard to all therapy clients and practitioners. I now recognize that such universal positivism, notwithstanding its humanistic appeal, is illogical.

As distasteful as it may be, there are certain persons who are undeserving of presumed goodness or an attribution of high esteem. It is a fact that many legal complaints filed against practitioners are based on clients' pathology, lies, and criminality. Amongst practitioners, there are a few "bad apples." Unfortunately, the few errant practitioners have contributed greatly to the exaggerated criticisms and accountability measures directed at all practitioners by consumers and governmental regulators.

From my legal experience, I have come to recognize—and I believe that every practitioner should recognize—that therapists, despite the extent and nature of their training, are just as vulnerable as any other person to bad judgments and wrongdoing. By acknowledging the reality of the matter, hopefully there can be movement toward improved judgments and proper conduct by therapists. Also, forewarned by information about legal safeguards, hopefully they can better defend against unjustified and wrongful allegations from clients. This book offers safeguards.

Of critical importance, it is hereby underscored that, without exception, every answer to a question in this book is intended for educational purposes only, and is not the rendering of legal opinion per se. Moreover, every answer, again without exception, is subject to modification or redefinition by the laws that are unique to the jurisdiction(s) in which the reader/practitioner provides professional services. It is essential that competent and qualified legal counsel familiar with the laws of the particular jurisdiction be obtained before deriving an idiosyncratic determination. As the reader progresses through the material, this caveat applies, as though repeated in full, to each and every question and answer.

Also, it must be recognized that the most subtle nuance of a scenario or situation could change the legal answer. Therefore, the reader is cautioned to avoid overgeneralization. Again, competent legal counsel is advised.

I wish to express appreciation to my law clients for affording me the opportunity to share in their practices, from dilemmas to exultations. One of the best rewards of being an attorney has been the connections formed with mental health practitioners and learning from their ventures.

R. H. W.
Omaha, NE, and
Tallahassee, FL

1

Standard of Care and Negligence

By definition, in order to benefit society, a professional must provide high-quality services. Consequently, a substandard practice is potentially unprofessional. Since society created the concept of professionalism and deems it a privilege (rather than a right), the practitioner who fails to perform at an acceptable standard will be subject to censure.

For a period of time, mental health practitioners were allowed to police themselves via monitoring provided by professional associations. Within a particular professional association, an ethics committee would receive complaints and take actions to rectify the situation. Today, ethics committees are to be found in the American Psychological Association, the National Association of Social Workers, the American Association for Marriage and Family Therapy, the American Counseling Association, and the American Psychiatric Association.

Since the action taken by an ethics committee against the errant practitioner was carried out by colleagues, all too often consumers found it to be insufficient. By the mid-1970s, more

1

and more complainants began to take legal action against professionals, including mental health practitioners. For about the last
two decades, the number of malpractice lawsuits against health
care professionals, again including mental health practitioners,
has escalated.

Malpractice or professional liability lawsuits are based on
negligence theory. The plaintiff (e.g., a therapy client) must set
forth a cause(s) of action, alleging that the defendant (e.g., a
mental health practitioner) has breached the standard of care.

To be liable, the defendant must owe the plaintiff a duty to
maintain or avoid a certain kind of conduct. Note that conduct
can occur by omission or commission. Within the therapist–client
relationship, this duty is clear-cut.

Whatever the allegedly wrongful conduct, the plaintiff must
suffer injury, with a causative nexus or connection between the
defendant's conduct and the injury. There must be proof that
the cause of action, say infliction of intentional emotional distress,
actually occurred in a manner that was outside the professional
standard of care. The breach of the standard of care must cause
an injury to the plaintiff and be attributable to the defendant's
conduct. Further, the injury must be compensable; that is, money
is used to restore the injured person (obviously, it is compensation, not restoration, that actually occurs). Under certain circumstances, and in some jurisdictions, the amount of the monetary
judgment can go beyond the injury, and include punitive damages intended to teach a lesson to other practitioners in the profession.

By distinction, while malpractice lawsuits require proof of
injury and that compensation is possible, complaints to ethics
committee or governmental regulatory agencies (e.g., licensing
boards) can result in sanctions for certain conduct by a practitioner that did not create injury per se. In other words, it is a
punitive discipline intended both to punish the wrongdoer and
serve notice on members of the professional discipline that such
conduct is unacceptable. Usually the penalties imposed by ethics
committees and regulatory agencies are intended to also safeguard society, or other consumers, from further wrongdoing by
the defendant or other practitioners.

Within the therapeutic relationship, identifying a specific and singular standard of care that is applicable to a particular set of circumstances, is difficult more often than not. The reason is simple: each set of circumstances must yield an idiosyncratic definition of the standard(s) to maintain; and there are no preordained or defining criteria that pinpoint exactly what must or must not occur in mental health services.

In general, the term *standard of care* refers to the qualities and conditions that prevail or should prevail in the particular mental health service. The qualitative assessment will be determined by what a reasonable and prudent practitioner in like circumstances would do.

The fact that the profession does not specify certain qualities and conditions is not justification for conduct. It is possible for an entire profession to fail to adopt or support qualities and conditions that society, by public policy and laws, would deem mandatory and to be scrupulously honored by the profession as a whole. For example, if a certain diagnostic or screening procedure (e.g., psychological testing) could be inexpensively administered to assure a substantially elevated intervention (i.e., a more efficacious form of therapy), public policy would support its provision, notwithstanding the fact that the profession had not embraced the idea; and liability could ensue for any and all members of the profession. To establish what a profession should be supporting becomes a matter of evaluating the expense of a given act or service, the concomitant risks, the possible invasiveness to personal rights, and the social conscionability—and then balancing these assessments against the possible benefits to the individual and society.

Any service must be predicated on theoretical and technical ideas that are held by a substantial portion of the relevant profession. Thus, practicing according to a theoretical model that is not within a recognized "school" of thought in the profession would likely fail to reach the requisite standard. Public policy tends not to support unbridled innovation, although this is clearly an avenue for possibly advancing knowledge and enhancing professional services.

In this day and age, the practitioner has less authority for idiosyncratic preferences in professional services. That is, today's mental health practitioner is greatly constrained by laws, and restricted to fewer and fewer individual judgments vis-à-vis assessment and intervention strategies. Because of public skepticism about health care in general, and, some would say, mental health services in particular, prescriptions and proscriptions are proliferating. Professional associations, striving to recover the previously elevated status that was stripped from them in the 1970s, are disseminating positions statements, commonly termed *guidelines* or *standards*, and revising ethics codes to be more specific. But of greater controlling power, state regulatory agencies, associated with the licensing boards for the mental health specialties, are promulgating statutes and rules that micromanage clinical decision making. The prescriptions and proscriptions, along with the actions taken by the rejuvenated ethics committees in professional associations and the burgeoning power accorded to regulatory agencies, often contribute support for malpractice legal actions.

The foregoing provides a basic introduction the scope of this chapter. The questions and answers in this chapter will explain and explore a variety of principles relevant to negligence and standard of care. The practice situations revealed in the questions will clarify how the mental health professional must continually process issues of standard of care and negligence.

I practice my own brand of therapy. I disagree with the idea that there are certain standards that have to be maintained by all therapists. If I believe that I am doing good therapy, why should I have to be subject to the opinions of other sources?

Being an intelligent, educated professional, it is not surprising that a therapist has the ability to create his or her own brand of therapy. It may well be superior to other forms of treatment. The therapist chooses, however, to accept "professional" status.

The cloak of professionalism is awarded by society. While the practitioner has earned the right to potentially wear the cloak, he or she can never own the vestment outright. Stated most directly:

Professionalism is not a right, it is a privilege. While a person earns the mantle by "paying dues," such as receiving a graduate degree and/or passing a licensing examination, continuing as a professional requires such things as adhering to standards of professional practice.

Public policy—an amorphous combination of beliefs, attitudes, mores, values, ethics, and laws—provides the basis for determining acceptable therapeutic practices. While the individual therapist has an opportunity to justify, say, a unique approach to treatment, it must be judged and approved by other sources. Thus, research-based communications will be necessary for scholarly peer review. This means that other well-credentialed therapists must potentially agree that a particular type of treatment is consonant with the standards for the academic discipline.

By law, negligence theory proscribes a therapist's being on a "frolic of his or her own," and prescribes that, to manifest an acceptable standard of care, the therapist must follow a "school" of thought or therapy that is recognized and endorsed by a substantial portion of pertinent professionals.

There is reason to believe that any approach to therapy is potentially subject to comparison, such as in a professional malpractice case, to rather traditional—yes, even conservative—treatment approaches. Because, while society wants to encourage innovation as a means for accommodating advances in knowledge and practice, it will not tolerate foolish experimentation with undue risks to consumers (formerly termed *clients* or *patients*). If there is a challenge to the acceptability of a therapeutic school, it is common for the plaintiff to rely on traditional voices to tell the trier of fact (i.e., the judge or the jury) what would be the safest and most acceptable treatment routes. Often the voices are quite conservative. While the traditional, prudent, and conservative viewpoint may dampen enthusiasm for innovations which might potentially lead to new benefits for the consumer and society, it also provides safeguards for consumers and society by setting a rather stringent test for treatment approaches in order to weed out unscientific, illogically formulated, and unproven ideas about therapy.

All therapists need not practice the same treatment approach, but they must all be prepared to justify their preferences for practices. Self-determination is inadequate; professional peer review is essential. Even then, there must be a meshing with other treatment modalities, or else the risk of legal liability is elevated.

Why should the therapist be subject to the opinions of others? The answer is simple. The therapist has chosen to be deemed a "professional," with all the benefits that are "attendant thereto" (to use a bit of legal jargon). If the therapist wants to dance the professional tune, he or she must be willing to pay the public policy piper.

I belong to no professional associations. Am I correct in thinking that I still have to abide by the code of ethics for the main association for my discipline?

There is no requirement per se that a therapist must honor the code of ethics promulgated by a professional association for which he or she is not a dues-paying member. Generally, the law views a professional association as a social organization, one that may be incorporated as a nonprofit corporation (though to enjoy this status, there are many restrictions on activities, such as using funds for political purposes).

Further, the diminution of status extends from health care practitioners to their professional associations. For example, recall how the Clinton Administration rejected requests from the American Medical Association (AMA) to be part of the inner circle planning health care reform, with the rebuke being essentially, "the AMA does not belong in government, it is just a special interest lobbying group."

There are some jurisdictions that allow the relevant professional association a limited degree of special input into the legal formulations pertaining to the discipline; for example, in statutes to which the association's code of ethics is relevant. However, part of the mission of the Federal Trade Commission (FTC) is to prevent monopolies taking control of society and the government, whether they are profit or nonprofit corporations. This prevents any professional association having unilateral authority over a discipline. Nonetheless, some states do have statutes that make reference to standards set by professional associations.

Certainly a professional association can, and should, have influence over members of a discipline, such as publishing lists of therapists licensed by the state to provide services to the public. Numerous courts of law and state licensing sources have supported professional associations' position statements, such as via a code of ethics, but only for the purpose of guiding the court or state agency in its deliberations and determinations. As one chair of a state licensing board said: "When we are adjudicating a licensing complaint case, we are aware of what the [association relevant to therapy] says in its code of ethics, but we never allow that to be the whole story—we consider it as but a part of many views, not the least of which is what we believe is best for our constituents."

Therefore, being a member of a professional association, and being subject to its code of ethics, is not mandatory for being a good professional. On the other hand, if the therapist ever faces a legal complaint, such as from a licensing board, being able to point out that he or she has, in fact, adhered to the code of ethics or other standards promulgated by, say, the most prestigious national mental health association aligned with his or her discipline and practice will typically provide a useful defense.

I believe being a "specialist" reflects status and will increase my earning potential. Is this wise legally?

Claiming to be a "specialist" has a seductive appeal, but it may be attractive for the wrong reasons. Commonly, it is believed that being a specialist will attract consumers for services. The person in need of a therapist will believe that the specialist has greater skill than other therapists in the community for the particular type of therapy or problem. Thus, it is reasoned, the consumer will prefer and purchase the services of a specialist, as opposed to those of a generalist.

Unfortunately, some therapists get a bit carried away, and claim to be a specialist without actually acquiring superior or refined skills. Also, some therapists proclaim competency in multiple specialties. This may backfire. As one consumer said, "When

I saw how many specialties that therapist advertised in the yellow pages of the telephone directory, I knew that no one person could be highly skilled in so many things, so I looked for another therapist.''

If a legal action occurs, the standard of care that will be imposed will usually be elevated for the professional claiming to be a specialist. For example, the defendant therapist might have to prove to the court that he or she provided services with competency greater than, say, that possessed by other therapists in the community. Indeed, it might be that the standard recognized by the court would be derived from a national level credentialing process for specialists with which the therapist had no actual affiliation. In other words, claiming to be a specialist will often result in an elevated standard of care being necessary, which can lead to the imposition of specific qualifications and competencies that are well beyond the therapist's professional background.

In this litigious era, there is ample justification for believing that understatement, rather than overstatement, provides the legally safe haven coveted by prudent therapists. Also, while ''puffing'' the quality of a widget might increase the sale of the product, there is no incontrovertible research to support that holding oneself out as a specialist will assuredly lead to a stronger therapeutic business. With the escalation of managed health care, there is, in fact, reason to believe that specialization will produce fewer economic rewards. The Clinton Administration, managed health care, and health insurance companies have made it patently clear through policies and payment arrangements that elevated specialist status will not be rewarded.

Whenever there is an inclination to claim to be a specialist, business planning strategies should be used to determine the potential therapeutic marketplace payoff. In turn, the business analysis should be interfaced with risk management goals; that is, how being a specialist will (or will not) create additional risk of, say, a malpractice or licensing complaint. Finally, consideration should be given to how much ego or self-aggrandizement may be underlying the idea of being a specialist. Nonetheless, there will, of course, be times when specialization is wise by all criteria, and then, but only then, the move to specialization should be made.

I consider myself a specialist in a certain kind of therapy, but I am basically self-taught and have no certifications, except my general license to practice. Do I have any unusual legal risk?

Refer back to the first question in this section, and note how the answer pointed out the need to receive approval from the profession. When a professional tries to practice a specialization that is without peer sanction, he or she will practice with peril.

Great caution should always be exercised. Depending on the nature of the special kind of treatment, it is best to construct an academic rationale, buttressed by empirical research. Preferably the therapist's theory, techniques, and research should be in writing and eventually published in a scholarly journal or book by a legitimate publishing source, not by a "vanity press." At the very least, the therapist should be prepared to present his or her ideas to other therapists at professional meetings, thereby orienting other practitioners in a manner that will lead to their being supportive rather than oppositional. Keep in mind that the standard of care, especially if it is the therapist's own creation, and particularly if he or she is self-taught, like all therapeutic services in this health care reform era, will be held to stringent legal accountability.

Finally, under managed health care there is the possibility that unique treatment modalities may not be reimbursed. Granted, this may not be logical, but funding treatment is still a condition controlled by the health care system, and, innovation and an extended array of services are not prized.

As I start to treat a client, I avoid forming any diagnostic opinions. In fact, I believe the concept of diagnosis is wrong and could create a barrier to psychological growth. I prefer to take the client's psychological ball and together we will start unraveling the lifestrings. However, I keep hearing about treatment planning. Since I know what I am doing, can I forget about this treatment planning stuff?

Among the humanists and phenomenologists, particularly in the 1960s and 1970s, there was a belief that diagnosis led to judgments that contradicted facilitative therapeutic conditions. Similarly, it was believed that it was best to allow the client to progress gradually, at a self-determined pace. In fact, it was thought that direction to the inner core by the therapist would, like diagnosis, contradict effective therapy.

Rightly or wrongly, times have changed. Today, public policy, which dictates the law, holds that therapy must be academically and scientifically based. Also, the prevailing view is that treatment must be carefully tailored to the needs unique to the particular consumer, which means having an individualized treatment plan. Certainly managed health care systems predicate financial reimbursement on well-formulated treatment plans.

While a licensing statute or a related rule may not state specifically that the therapist must have an individualized treatment plan, there is reason to believe that the standard of care, which is always nebulous and evolving, embraces both diagnosis and individualized treatment planning. Prosecuting attorneys, who are certainly not therapists, have been known to assert that their analyses of licensing complaint cases always look early on for a clear-cut diagnosis, aligned with the DSM-IV (or some similar nosological system recognized by the overall field of mental health), and a subsequent treatment plan that is tailored to the consumer's needs. They also look for proof, such as in the treatment notes, that the therapist has followed the individualized treatment plan, monitored it for effectiveness, and made changes as merited.

The incongruence between humanistic therapy and current legal concepts has led some plaintiff-attorneys to say, in effect, "Whenever I do a deposition with a therapist and he or she admits to being humanistic, I rejoice because I know that it is unlikely that the therapist can justify his or her treatment in terms acceptable to a judge or jury, which means it is most likely that my client will prevail."

The foregoing antithetical stance may seem unfair to humanistic therapy, but it exists and must be reckoned with by every humanistically oriented therapist. The way to counter an attack on humanistic therapy is to construct an academic rationale and be able to articulate it in clear-cut and concrete terms. Esoteric, vague, head-in-the-clouds ideas are inadequate, and it is easy to succumb to the "feel good" nature of humanistic therapy, as opposed to buckling down and being academically prepared for the standards imposed by public policy and the law.

As for "unraveling the lifestrings" from the consumer's ball, forget it. The notions of diagnosis and individualized treatment planning mean that therapeutic interventions must be purposeful. While humanistic theory supports the client's being responsible for choosing the therapeutic trail, the modern public policy and managed health care views are that therapist must be the trail boss, determining each step along the path toward long-term objectives and short-term therapeutic goals that have been identified and monitored by professional skills.

Since I know that certain situations require psychological tests, such as for justifying payment from a health insurance company or to make my courtroom testimony sound really "expert," I often administer a whole batch of tests. I must, however, confess that I do not always score tests, at least not all of them. And sometimes I will use my own short form. Given that I rely primarily on my clinical impressions and judgments based on what the client says to me in interviews, the test results, even though not strictly by the book in the way they were administered, seem to fulfill their purpose. Do you think that this is okay?

The foregoing question presents several issues that are problematic. There are three pronounced clues of high-risk conduct:

First, to administer "a whole batch of tests" and then not truly use them for the benefit of the consumer is to leave the therapist exposed to all sorts of liability, from the health insurance company, the consumer, or a licensing board. Stated bluntly, the therapist's conduct would be subject to being branded a scheme for unjust enrichment, and certainly not in accord with professional standards, managed health care policies, or laws.

Second, if put to an ethical or a legal analysis (e.g., litigation involving the therapist), the standard of care, without doubt, would consider how well any psychological test fulfilled the qualities promulgated by professional authorities. There are, of course, well-accepted standards for educational and psychological tests, which include prescriptions for, among other things, reliability and validity. Use of one's "own short form" without the under-pinnings of professional standards could be viewed as negligence.

Third, "clinical impressions and judgments" are appropriate and essential, but are not sufficient; they are part of all therapy, but they must complement, not replace, more formal and stan-dardized assessment methods. Professionalism will not sanction an excursion beyond the realm of recognized standards for psy-chological testing.

It is my understanding that, if I have another therapist endorse the way that I am treating a particular client, this will eliminate the possibility of any complaint about my treatment approach. Is this correct?

There would be great comfort from finding a single action that would eliminate the possibility of any complaint about a treat-ment approach. Alas and alack, there is no such panacea. Having another therapist endorse the treatment approach is, however, a step in the right direction. As discussion of supervision in the next two questions and answers will reveal, supervision is an important source of protection against legal problems.

In seeking endorsement from another therapist, the purpose is to show that peer review was obtained and the treatment ap-proach was in accord with standards maintained by the profes-sional discipline (or a significant portion thereof). Thus, the review and subsequent endorsement should be sought from a mainline, noncontroversial colleague, consultant, or supervisor. As might be expected, the more formal his or her credentials, the more solid his or her professional reputation, and the more objective the nature of the relationship between the supervisor and the supervisee (i.e., no undue favoring of the supervisee), the greater will be the benefit for risk management for the thera-pist (and quality care for the consumer).

I want to make use of supervision, but do not want to incur the expense of paying another therapist. Can a colleague and I swap supervisory services, that is, supervise each other's cases?

For quality care for the consumer and risk management for the therapist, it is axiomatic that every therapist, regardless of how

many years that he or she has been in practice, should have supervision in some form. It is foolhardy to believe that years of experience or financial cost negate the need for supervision.

The penultimate rule is "any supervision is better than no
supervision." The ultimate rule is "the more expert and objective
the supervision, the better."

Yes, the therapist can receive supervision from any other professional who has relevant expertise. Yes, the therapists could
"swap services." As should be evident (in this answer and the
next question and answer as well), swapping services may be a
faulty or less than ideal plan.

While payment per se is not the sine qua non of supervision,
it obviously attests to a professional relationship. What payment
signifies is, of course, some degree of motivation on the part of
the supervisor or consultant that goes beyond friendship with
the supervisee.

The wisest approach is to accept that mental health practice
exists in a litigious society, and one of the essential costs of doing
business in this era is to have legal and quality care safeguards,
as cultivated by supervision. Having a formal supervisory relationship is certainly worth the financial expenditure. Remember the
old adages "you get what you pay for" and "an ounce of prevention is worth a pound of cure."

**What is the best way to structure supervision to minimize any
legal risks?**

The greatest legal protection will come from having a formal
supervisory relationship with a supervisor who has strong credentials and professional stature. The supervisory sessions should be
formal and structured, and progress notes should be made. Ide-
ally, the supervisor should have access to all cases being treated
by the therapist-supervisee. Bringing in "only problem cases" re-
duces the legal protection. The sessions should follow a set
schedule.

Alternatively, it is possible, as mentioned earlier, to receive
some legal protection via supervision from virtually any other professional with relevant expertise, but this is a less desirable course.

Having a colleague or a business associate review cases is better than nothing. Even here, efforts should be made to maintain formalities and structure, such as having sessions on a regular basis and with records of the supervision being maintained.

It is important to recognize that the supervisor will incur liability for the cases that he or she reviews, or, given the circumstances, should have reviewed. Therefore, being a supervisor carries a legal risk. In one case, the therapist agreed to a former trainee's use of the therapist's name as "supervisor" on various documents. When a patient filed a lawsuit against the "supervisee," the supervisor (who had not actually provided supervision) was, nonetheless, held to have liability and ended up paying a substantial sum of money in damages to the plaintiff.

I am a practical person, and hate to spend a buck if it can be avoided. A number of other therapists in the community have brochures and other materials that seem to give pizzazz to their practice. I suspect that they have these printed to try to create an elevated impression of themselves. Should I have a brochure of some sort?

Yes, having a brochure or some form of client information about the policies and other matters that govern and influence the mental health services is an excellent idea. These materials should not, however, be thought of as being primarily for "pizzazz" or promotion.

The primary purpose of a service brochure is risk management, that is, having materials that orient the consumer to professional qualifications and policies (e.g., about financial responsibilities), relationship boundaries, and create a quasi-contractual framework for the service.

It is good to have an established routine, as could be attested to by office personnel, that every consumer (and perhaps his or her significant others) receives the orientation materials upon initial entry for treatment. The consumer could, of course, sign an acknowledgement of having received the materials, but if there is a definite routine that the therapist and others can attest to having been maintained, signatures end up being helpful but not mandatory.

Again, the primary purpose of the service brochure is not promotional, it is to set forth the "rules" for being a consumer of the therapist's professional services. This provides a definition for what the consumer could reasonably expect in the way of standards or other legal considerations.

To save money, I am thinking about having my office in my home. However, I have a house full of kids, and I can foresee a different atmosphere from the one I now have in a professional building. Is there any legal issue about a home office that I should consider?

There is no reason to automatically avoid a home office, but the question identifies some trouble spots. Kids will be kids, and therapy must be therapy. One of the most obvious considerations is the contemporary press for a therapist to keep his or her personal and professional life well separated.

The boundary of the professional relationship can become blurred by normal household events interfering with treatment conditions. While it might seem philosophically desirable to allow a consumer to witness the healthy home relationship enjoyed by the therapist, it is not consonant with prudent mental health practice in this day and age. There have been legal cases wherein a client who welcomed, even encouraged, being seen at the therapist's home office ended up alleging that he or she was wrongfully seduced into coming to the home as a way of abusing the treatment relationship.

Paying overhead for an office in a professional building is often thought of as financially draining, and the extra room at the house with a private entrance may seem enticing. For both quality care for the client and legal protection for the therapist, a decision to see consumers in a home office should be carefully evaluated. In general, it is certainly less desirable, all things being equal, than having an office in a professional building.

I have an unlisted home telephone. If a client wants to reach me after hours, it is necessary to call my answering service, and I call them back when it is convenient. Several clients have objected to not being able to call me directly. Should I make my home number available to clients?

There are good reasons for not allowing consumers to telephone the therapist at home. There is always the boundary issue; the therapist's personal life must be kept separate from his or her professional life.

No matter what the justification by either the consumer or the therapist, the consumer must not be allowed into the therapist's personal life. There have been lawsuits that involved the consumer-litigant's alleging the therapist "told me that I was special, not just a client, she even gave me her unlisted home telephone and told me to call anytime." While the consumer may be exaggerating or even fabricating, the circumstances may be interpreted legally as pointing toward unprofessional conduct. In this era of doubt about health care providers, this type of allegation might be difficult to turn aside.

There is also the issue of allowing a consumer to gain reinforcement for an unhealthy motive. For example, accommodating a demand from a consumer that he or she be allowed to have the therapist's unlisted telephone number is potentially reinforcing an unhealthy dependence, which potentially could work against important therapeutic goals. Also, it would certainly remove control from the therapist and place it with the consumer. The therapist must always control every aspect of the professional relationship; otherwise, liability will escalate.

Finally, assuming that unhealthy reinforcement could be avoided and therapeutic control could be retained, allowing consumers to telephone the therapist at home can have a disruptive impact on the therapist's family members. If they suffer, the therapist suffers; and if the therapist suffers, the consumers suffer.

I have an outpatient psychotherapy practice. I am concerned about the possibility that one of my clients might have an emergency, say a suicide attempt, and need to reach me quickly. At the same time, I want to maintain a reasonable personal life—heaven knows that my work already creates impositions on my family members, what with my always returning calls and filling out insurance forms at home. Must I have a beeper so that any client can reach me any time, any place?

No, the therapist does not necessarily have to carry a beeper. Indeed, the therapist does not necessarily have to be available for emergencies.

From the first professional contact with a client (and any significant others who are involved), the therapist should make it patently clear that he or she does not assure availability at all times and the practice is not geared to the provision of emergency services. Instead, the therapist should inform all concerned that, in case of a psychiatric emergency and the therapist not being readily available to assist them in making arrangements, immediate contact should be made with an appropriate emergency facility in the community.

It is good practice to supply all clients with the names and addresses of several emergency services. Also, a therapist should seek a special arrangement or affiliation with a primary emergency service, such as a psychiatric hospital, which would yield a clear-cut contact plan that can be communicated to all clients at the onset of treatment. Incidentally, it is always best to have established a personal relationship with emergency and other referral sources, thereby paving the way for clients to gain access, as well as keeping the therapist in the service plan.

An important legal principle centers on the client having no reasonable basis for believing that the therapist stands ready to intervene on an emergency basis. Certain emergencies will require family members or significant others to help the client locate and enter an emergency program. Thus, the information should be made available to all those having caregiving or supportive roles with the client. Of course, confidentiality or privileged communication dictate that the transmission of this information be done with the client's approval. Whenever possible, it is advisable to have the client transmit the information, and verify, such as by a written statement, that all interested parties have been informed and understand the emergency system.

Finally, the therapist is wise to want to preserve his or her home life. To a large extent, effectiveness as a therapist hinges upon personal physical and mental health. Personal rights, such as the right to privacy, must be honored. The therapist's family is entitled to be free from undue disruptions caused by professional factors. Therefore, drawing lines for the therapist's availability is essential, providing that other arrangements for clients have been made that will reasonably meet their needs.

Our outpatient psychotherapy office closes on weekends. While we do have an answering service, it is common for my two partners and myself to travel or be unavailable. Should we purposely schedule ourselves so that one of us is always readily available, in other words, to be "on call?"

The preceding question and answer applies to this situation. As a supplement, if the therapist has created a reasonable expectation in the mind of the client that weekend telephone calls will receive a response, it likely will be necessary to have a therapist on call.

When partner-therapists become involved with each other's clients, each is in the service chain and faces potential legal liability. Therefore, several preventive steps should be taken, such as having an acknowledgement from each client that another partner-therapist has a limited right to know their confidential or privileged information and the partner-therapists maintain ongoing supervision of each other's cases to assure the appropriate standard of care.

An alternative is to communicate to all clients and their significant others that, since it is an outpatient psychotherapy practice and not open on the weekends, any weekend emergencies should be directed to a psychiatric emergency service in the community, as discussed in the preceding question and answer. Remember that the legal principle involves what the client has a reasonable basis for believing to be the therapist's service duty. If the therapist educates the client to the therapist's and his or her partners' not being available on weekends, and that psychiatric emergencies should be directed to another source (i.e., a community emergency service), it will lessen legal risks considerably and justify the therapist and the professional partners pursuing healthy personal life-styles on weekends.

Remember the old adage: "Some people live to work, while other people work to live." Surely the therapist should prefer keeping work in perspective.

2

The Company You Keep

Collegiality is a primary aspect of professionalism. The promotion of the profession, with all the benefits that can accrue to society, is thought to best occur by pooling the knowledge and expertise of colleagues. Stated differently, professionals should come together as peers, and work collaboratively to advance the discipline.

As will be recalled from the preceding chapter, society at one time gave deference to collegial monitoring of errant practitioners by allowing ethics committees to protect the rights, interests, and welfare of society. Of course, this deference was eliminated by the shift in public policy which revealed dissatisfaction with peer discipline, and a new era of governmental regulation and malpractice litigation was born.

Regrettably, many mental health practitioners seem to cling to an illogical, out-dated notion that collegiality should pervade all spheres of professional functioning. Letting collegiality dominate in an age in which control is actually vested in legal sources, can have devastating effects, such as inept business operations, faulty judgments about clinical strategies, and unnecessary legal risks. Parenthetically, this irrational clinging to collegiality is commonly attributable to misinformation being disseminated by professors in academia. Divorced from the real world of practice and being advocates of professional associations, the professors of this ilk pursue aggrandizement of the institutionalized organization. For example, any source that asserts, explicitly or implicitly, that the preferences of the academy or a professional association are superior to legal dictates is foolish and creates a potential risk for the individual member.

Perhaps the greatest pitfall created by blind allegiance to collegiality is vicarious liability. In this age of elevated professional liability, two or more colleagues involved in a shared enterprise, such as being in practice together, have the risk of being liable for the other's conduct. Through its laws, society asserts that each person in a shared enterprise, since each benefits from the consortium (e.g., financially), has a duty to exercise reasonable and diligent effort to safeguard the public or consumers from his or her associates' wrongdoing. From the legal perspective, one bad apple can spoil the whole basket; that is, one practitioner's wrongdoing can extend legal liability to the others in the practice group.

Today, collegiality does not include total tolerance. The concept of "peer" can no longer be exempt from being tested and monitored. While there is equality between affiliated practitioners, the equality has its limits. Constant vigilance, perhaps even healthy suspicion, can assure that all affiliates are meeting the standard of care.

This chapter delves into the legal implications of being in a practice with others. The commitment to quality care will be discussed in the context of legal mandates and business principles. The prudent professional will discover that affiliations are inextricably intertwined with clinical, business, and legal principles. Later chapters will elaborate further on this matter.

I have considerable turnover of employees. My secretarial and clerical employees tend to come and go. Sometimes I even hire someone from a temporary service. It has dawned on me that these workers have access to the names of my clients and all sorts

of confidential information. What would happen if an employee revealed something confidential out in the community?

Since employees are agents of the therapist, the therapist has potential legal liability for the conduct of the employees who breach confidentiality. To minimize the risk of liability, the therapist *must* provide all employees with reasonable training and supervision to assure that confidentiality is maintained, whether in or out of the office. From the onset, all applicants for employment should be carefully screened for their seeming ability to fulfill the objective of confidentiality. Once a person is hired, he or she should be schooled in policies about maintaining confidentiality during and after employment with the therapist.

A written agreement with the employee is a good idea. It should specify how the information should be safeguarded, and the employee should acknowledge being trained, and pledge to uphold conditions that protect confidentiality.

If the therapist has made a reasonable effort to select, train, and supervise employees for the maintenance of confidentiality, a breach by an ex-employee could still be problematic; but the therapist would have an appropriate defense and might well be exonerated. By accepting a position with an implicit or explicit contractual condition to maintain confidentiality, the breaching employee, even though he or she is not a professional per se, could be held legally accountable.

It should be added that confidentiality is just one of many conditions that merit coverage in personnel management. Every employee must be prepared to protect and promote the clients' best interests.

I am one of three therapists. We are equal owners of an incorporated clinic. Since we are all senior therapists, we have little to do with each other's cases. When we meet, we usually just talk about business issues, like expenditures for operating the office. If one of my colleagues should be sued for malpractice or have a licensing complaint filed against him or her, do I have any possible legal risk?

If professionals are engaged in a shared enterprise, such as being co-owners of a mental health clinic, there is a distinct possibility

that each of them could be potentially liable for the negligence of
another of them. Under public policy, receiving therapy services
involving multiple professionals has a reasonable basis for believing that all members of the clinic should be exercising efforts
to assure that standards are met for safeguarding the consumers.
After all, a shared enterprise provides each owner with revenues
or other benefits from the association.

At issue here is the legal principle of vicarious liability. Even
though a professional does not commit a damaging act, his or her
affiliation with and the benefits derived from the alleged offender
justify liability. By public policy and law, negligence is imputed
to all concerned with operating the professional service or clinic.

Incidentally, the long-established common law principle of
master-servant imposes vicarious liability on the senior practitioner (i.e., the employer or "master") for the conduct of the
junior practitioner (i.e., the employee or "servant").

Incidentally, if there are multiple senior practitioners, they
could have joint and several liability, meaning that they could be
held collectively or individually responsible. Moreover, for multiple defendants, the damages could be proportional or dispropor-
tional, the latter meaning that one therapist might be ordered to
pay more than another therapist. This particular issue is determined by the laws of the individual state jurisdiction.

Tort theory accepts that an injured person must be protected
and compensated for damages inflicted upon him or her by a
servant. Since a negligent servant (i.e., the tort-feasor) commonly
has minimal financial resources, the liability for making payment
to the injured person is imputed to the master who is presumed
to be more financially able. Historically, it has been clear-cut that
the rationale was monetary; that is, intended to allow an injured
litigant to reach the "deep pocket" for financial compensation
for damages. Currently, this notion is alive and well, and certainly
applicable to mental health practice.

**If I rent space on an hourly basis to a therapist, do I have any
liability for alleged malpractice on the part of the other therapist?**

Rental arrangements may or may not involve vicarious liability.
The primary test is probably what the consumer could reasonably

assume from the cues in the context in which the services are provided. For example, if a singular clinic name is used for the practice and the consumer has a reasonable basis for believing that the practitioners in the clinic are associated, there might be vicarious liability. But if the therapists studiously present their practices as being independent (e.g., separate letterhead stationary, billings, listings in the yellow pages, etc.), the possibility of vicarious liability would be much less.

I own a mental health practice and need to have an associate. I do not, however, want to be legally liable for the associate's services. If I refer to the associate as an "independent contractor," as opposed to an "employee," can I avoid liability for his or her malpractice?

In and of itself, the title used for an associate or contractual arrangement agreed upon between the senior therapist and the associate will not determine whether or not vicarious liability exists. Again, the basic test is what could the consumer reasonably assume? If there is an indication that the consumer can reasonably assume that each practitioner has a watch-dog or quality-care responsibility to safeguard clients, the liability would not be circumvented by title or contract.

Another therapist and I rent an office suite together. Occasionally we refer a patient to one another, or I might do therapy and my suite mate might do the psychological testing with the same patient. Do we have any liability for each other?

There is never an indelible demarcation for vicarious liability. Generally, if there is a referral to another professional for supplemental services, there is not automatic liability imposed on the professional who implemented the referral. Of course, it would be a different matter if the referring professional had a business relationship with the particular referral source, made use of no other referral sources for the supplemental service, gave the client no other option for receiving the supplemental service, or used strong persuasion (i.e., undue influence) to basically force the client to seek the supplemental services from the designated source.

Since this scenario describes the two practitioners as being located at the same site, the specter of liability is hovering in the background. Further, regardless of the proximity of the offices, an attorney analyzing the treatment situation for a client allegedly impacted upon by malpractice would likely evaluate, among other things, the acts committed or omitted by each practitioner in the chain of treatment. Thus, unless the malpractice was clearly from a singular source, the instant scenario would portend to impose liability on both practitioners, given that they both provided services to the client.

I have a partner who is also a therapist. My partner plays it straight in the office with clients, but I know that his or her personal life is rather wild and bordering on what some might think was criminal conduct. Let me be blunt—my partner engages in promiscuous sex and uses recreational drugs. It is obvious that there will be no changes made, so what can I do to protect my reputation and practice?

The most obvious answer is to completely sever the professional relationship with the partner. Certainly an individual is entitled to his or her personal preferences for life-style, including certain acts that may be frowned upon by other folks. Rightly or wrongly, professional status carries the obligation of having to maintain a life-style that is reasonably acceptable to society. Any criminal conviction would most surely have implications for maintaining licensure, not to mention having a negative impact on professional reputation, which could, of course, lead to diminished income potential.

As a partner or colleague of the professional whose personal life includes misconduct, there might even be vicarious liability for his or her professional activities. For example, public policy would hold that the implied duty to supervise or safeguard consumers that applies to shared enterprises would ordain that there be absolutely no support of illicit activity, wherever it might be manifested. There is a risk that "looking the other way" would be viewed as tacit acceptance or condonement. Of course, diminution of professional reputation due to personal life-style for one partner might reach to diminished financial factors for the other partners.

In this era of accountability and competition in health care, it is illogical to be associated with any person who lives in a manner that will jeopardize professional status. The legal, reputation, and financial spillover effects are just too costly to accommodate a libertarian attitude about the conduct of one's professional colleagues.

It should also be noted that some jurisdictions have laws that may require mandatory reporting of licensed health care providers who are impaired in their practices. Being associated with such an impaired practitioner without reporting could, in those jurisdictions, impose regulatory discipline on all associates. See the next question and answer for more details.

My partner has a significant alcohol abuse problem. What should I do?

As mentioned previously, some jurisdictions have legal requirements that a licensed practitioner knowing of professional misconduct or a health-related condition that impairs professional functioning, must notify a regulatory source. There is considerable diversity between jurisdictions on this matter.

Even if there is no mandatory reporting of the errant or impaired professional, there may be a legal proscription about giving any sort of support to that person's practice of the profession. In this instance, it would be wise to terminate any affiliation with the practitioner, aside from personal, friendly encouragement to seek treatment.

I would like to affiliate with another professional in my discipline, perhaps forming a partnership. From a legal point of view and aside from academic credentials, what personal qualities should I look for in a partner?

Obviously there needs to be mutual attractiveness and compatibility to a significant degree, which logically means values and interests that are consonant. Based on experience with problem

couplings, it seems that there should be full and complete disclosure of all relevant information. Much like keeping a secret from
a fiancé prior to marriage, failing to reveal critical information
between business or practice partners is a harbinger of professional abuse and divorce.

Three areas that seem especially important to reveal and assess for risk are: substance abuse (how much alcohol is truly con-
sumed); management of personal finances (has there ever been
a bankruptcy, how much is owed on high-interest credit cards);
and sexual relations (what is the tendency to get involved in problematic intimate relationships).

Of course, a strong global index can be gained from simply
knowing how successful the would-be partner has been in all personal and professional spheres in life (have there been divorces,
are his or her offspring on a positive track, how much income has
actually been earned to date, are there any maladaptive habits).

**I have discovered that one of my employees has been submitting
claims to health insurance companies for sessions that did not
occur. No patient or insurance company has detected the false
claims. I would prefer to say nothing about it, unless it is detected.
Of course, I am not to blame, so surely I do not have to report
my employee. Perhaps, for a period of time, I should just set
aside the money that I received from the false claims, putting it
into an account. Then if it is detected, say by an insurance company, I can point out how I was planning to return the money to
them. Is this a good way to handle it?**

This scenario gives reason to believe that there may well be both
civil and criminal liability for the employee and employer alike.
While there may not be a legal mandate to report the errant
employee, certainly the employer has a legal duty to operate a
business in an honest manner. By knowing about the fraud and
failing to correct the situation, the employer is becoming a party
to the wrongdoing.

Incidentally, and as mentioned earlier, some jurisdictions
now have, as part of the licensing law, a requirement that one
licensee's knowing about another licensee's wrongdoing creates

a duty to report—and failing to make the report can result in discipline of the licensee who did not take action. In the least, fraudulent billing for services would fail to meet the prevailing standards for the profession, and would be subject in these jurisdictions to mandatory reporting.

The notion of saying that putting money into an account to prepare to pay back monies owed upon detection seems silly or sociopathic, and does nothing more than add to the wrongdoing. Such a scheme would be demonstrably an admission of knowledge of the fraud.

Greed destroys. Certainly this sort of situation is problematic, and there is no trouble-free way out of it. Of course the initial source of the problem was the dishonest employee, and the employer cannot afford to join in any fraudulent practice.

What would be the best solution? Again, there are likely to be negatives with any solution, but following the honest route is certainly the honorable approach.

Honesty requires immediate action to rectify the situation, such as making a refund to the payment sources, and taking steps to be sure it does not happen again; for example, by terminating the employee. In fact, filing charges against the employee would be evidence that the employer does not, in any way, condone the fraud.

3

Client Management

The changing times for mental health practice mean that the traditional notion of letting clients be, more or less, self-determining is no longer viable or legally safe. Today, legal and third-party payment sources expect, rightly or wrongly, that the practitioner will be a provider of quality services in a way that is product oriented.

The mental health practitioner must provide consumers with a service delivery system and related techniques that derive from behavioral science research, and have established an efficacious system for meeting the needs of the service recipient. Managed health care certainly reflects the foregoing set. Also, regulatory agencies are known to look askance at a clinical record that does not reveal clear-cut benefits to the client.

Consequently, many of the tenets of the insight-oriented psychotherapies must be considered suspect, or perhaps even unwise or unacceptable. In the long run, this viewpoint may prove to be ill advised. Society may be "throwing out the baby with the bathwater"; that is, the quest for cost reduction and accountability may result in many useful and valuable treatment or service alternatives being cast aside, with a loss of benefits to consumers.

Of great concern, the therapeutic relationship, that special alliance between therapist and client, has been altered by the escalation of legal liability on the part of the practitioner. While earlier psychotherapeutic approaches, particularly those with a humanistic bent, endowed the client with almost unfettered personal responsibility for and determination of the unique composition of the therapeutic relationship, the specter of ethical, regulatory, and malpractice complaints makes such a stance totally foolish today. Rather, the modern practitioner is expected to exercise competence for determining how the intervention will be structured and implemented, and do so in consonance with the standards required by ethics and law.

This chapter will offer a reframing of the therapeutic relationship. Avoiding ethical and legal complaints against the therapist is as important as accomplishing treatment gains for the client. These two objectives cannot be separated.

I tend to accept everyone who contacts me for treatment. On occasion, I encounter clients with problems or pathologies for which I have little or no training for treatment. I need the income, so I hate to turn away any potential client. What is my solution?

If the therapist attempts to treat a problem, pathology, or type of client without adequate training and experience, the therapist is probably violating the principle of competency that underlies ethics and laws relevant to clinical practice. There is no room for equivocation: the therapist cannot provide services to any client without competency that is in accord with the prevailing standard of care for the profession. Just from the negligence theory point of view, attempting to treat a certain condition without assured competency is foolhardy and carries extreme risk of allegations for malpractice legal action, as well as the possibility of complaints to ethics committees and regulatory agencies.

While anyone can appreciate the need for income, incompetency carries a heavy pricetag. Whatever income is derived by this approach is miniscule compared to the financial and professional costs associated with providing services in an incompetent manner.

For the benefit of clients and the therapist's own risk management and legal protection, the therapist should never accept a client for service unless he or she is confident that the competency necessary to establish the requisite standard of care can be documented. Legally safe practice is unquestionably linked to being selective about clientele, matching each client's needs with the therapist's competency, and assessing the risk that the particular client poses in other ways as well (e.g., proneness to litigation, inability to pay for services, willingness to adhere to the treatment plan, and so on).

There is no simple solution. Most basically, the therapist needs to adopt a revised view about income being all-determining of the clientele. The therapist needs to adopt a risk management stance, meaning that he or she acknowledges the legal risks associated with accepting a client for treatment when the therapist has no competency to treat that person.

Incidentally, besides risk management for the therapist, referring a client to another practitioner for his or her quality care does not necessarily mean that the therapist is, in fact, losing income. There is reason to believe that for every referral made to another practitioner, there will likely be a reciprocal referral. While it would be inappropriate to make a promise of reciprocal referrals a prerequisite for referrals, it is acceptable to consider which referral source(s) among the array of qualified referral sources would, in turn, reciprocate with referral support.

It is really frustrating to have a client who will not do homework assignments or even try things that I recommend during therapy. How can I convince the client that what I prescribe has to be done?

Obviously the initial attempts should be based on reason and logic, framing the recommendations as being for the welfare of the client. That is, the client should be told that following therapeutic prescriptions or homework assignments is essential if he or she is to accomplish the treatment goals.

If reason fails to persuade and induce adherence, it may be necessary to move to a more firm approach, and emphatically

declare that the therapist's legal duty is to provide quality care in
the best interests of the client. The therapist has prescribed a
treatment plan that is in the best interests of the client. If the
client will not adhere to the treatment plan, the therapist is obligated by professional standards, and probably the law of the particular state, to cease to provide treatment—because to do
otherwise would not be in the best interests of the client.

It is important to realize that the therapist will incur legal
liability by continuing to treat a client who is, with the therapist's
knowledge, not benefiting from the therapist's treatments, even
if it is due to the client's nonadherence to the treatment plan.
Thus, for the therapist to continue on with the treatment, assuming the therapist has made a reasonable effort to bring the client
into compliance with the treatment plan, would likely be viewed
as a breach of the standard of care.

**I am uncomfortable with the mandatory reporting laws, such as
for child abuse, in my state. I feel I should be free to use my
judgment about a situation. For example, if a client tells me about
having abused a child, but, in my professional opinion, has made
a sincere commitment to treatment which should eliminate any
future abuse, I think I should be able to not report the abuse.
Can I make such a judgment, and if I do, knowing it is against
the law, could I end up in trouble even though my intentions
were honorable?**

Certainly the expressed beliefs on this matter have a solid basis
in psychological theory, but rightly or wrongly, they lack a solid
basis in the law. Professional ethics make it clear that the law is
supreme. State statutes and rules are clear-cut about the legal
duty for mandatory reporting. Therefore, it would be illogical to
defy the law, harboring any notion of professional righteousness.
Yes, even with honorable intention or a therapeutic rationale, the
therapist could "end up in trouble" for failing to adhere strictly
to the laws of the jurisdiction.

The laws of some states or jurisdictions allow a bit of leeway
for some instances of child abuse that has occurred in the past

to go unreported. This is, however, a complex matter. If the therapist has a child abuse situation for which reporting is questionable, the decision to report or not to report can only be made knowledgeably by getting a legal opinion. The decision must be based on law, not therapeutic preference.

This whole idea about warning about dangerousness to self or others seems to be counter to good psychotherapy practice. Unless there was a clear-cut threat with a specific intended victim, I doubt that predictions of dangerousness by me or any other therapist can be wholly accurate. I believe that whatever a client tells a therapist should be kept absolutely confidential. How do I reconcile my theoretical beliefs with the duty to warn?

The therapist here is right. No matter what the diagnostician's training or experience, there is never a freedom from doubt about the accuracy of a prediction of dangerousness or violence. Studies reveal that predicting dangerousness or violence is tenuous at best. Nonetheless, public policy, as implemented by statutes and common law rulings, holds that error should be made on the side of conservatism. That is, it seems that false positives (i.e., predicting dangerousness or violence when it will not or does not actually occur) are within acceptable public policy. Stated bluntly, the prevailing view is that protecting the public is more important than the rights and needs of the individual patient.

The current state of affairs vis-à-vis warnings of dangerousness can understandably produce dismay for the conscientious therapist. The line of duty to warn cases, starting with the well known *Tarasoff versus the California Board of Regents* (17 Cal. 3d 358 [1976]), seems to make it clear that providing optimum therapeutic conditions is secondary to safeguarding others from the client's potential dangerousness or violence. There are legal provisions for the therapist breaching confidentiality or privileged communication in order to issue such warnings. In fact, potentially the therapist will be liable legally if he or she does not issue a timely warning.

As for determining when a warning is necessary, it is important to study the cases on the duty to warn, and know, particularly, how the statutes and courts within the jurisdiction(s) in which the therapist practices have addressed the issues. Commonly, the warning must be made if there is a reasonable basis for the therapist's believing the violence of bodily harm to self or others is imminent. Also, it may be necessary to take steps to intervene, such as implementing involuntary commitment or notifying law enforcement sources. Often a jurisdiction will have prescriptions for notifying sources of dangerousness (note that jurisdictions differ on how the warning is to be made).

Each clinical case can, of course, have unique conditions, and the uniquenesses will have to be subjectively weighed for significance. In any event, the therapist should, from the onset of and throughout treatment, monitor for dangerousness. It is preferable to use a consistent and objective system; however, simply asking the client about suicide or violent ideation is useful. Whatever the type of data on the matter, careful notes should be entered into the record to document that the therapist made a reasonable effort to assess the client's propensity for violence or dangerousness.

Are some kind of clients more likely to file legal complaints than other kinds of clients?

The research on this matter is sparse and certainly not definitive. Among attorneys involved with defending mental health practitioners, conventional wisdom seems to be that any element of narcissism is a harbinger of litigation. Structurally, narcissism seems to be connected to such personality types as hysterics, psychopathic deviates, and sociopaths. When a patient in one of these diagnostic categories also has paranoid tendencies and/or a denial of responsibility for personal actions, the risk of blaming someone else for a negative lot in life is increased. Also, clients with a multiple personality are a high risk for complaints, as are parents who are involved in child custody, visitation, or abuse cases.

By this time, it is apparent that the above categories of client make up a large portion of most therapists' clienteles. In other words, it is impossible to be a therapist and not encounter clients with personality characteristics that will lead to complaining about the therapist. This is the nature of mental health services in this highly litigious era.

Of course, the client with the greatest likelihood of filing some sort of complaint against a therapist is the client who has been allowed to build up a deficit in payment for services. It is almost axiomatic that attempting to collect an overdue debt from a client is tantamount to inviting an ethical, regulatory, or malpractice complaint, no matter how clear-cut the debt.

4

Forensic Services

One of the most notable confirmations of the importance of the mental health professions is witnessed by mental health professionals being integral to the legal system.

While there is a myriad of legally related roles that a mental health practitioner can fulfill, one that carries high status is that of offering expert testimony in legal cases. As will be underscored later, being available to serve as an expert in legal cases has become an essential part of professionalism.

Providing forensic services may be welcomed or unwelcomed by the practitioner. Regardless of the nature of the particular legal role or forensic service, it is likely that practitioners providing forensic mental health services will experience the situation as being mentally complex, academically challenging and stimulating, and potentially rewarding in terms of finances and self satisfaction.

There is, however, a downside to providing forensic services. The expectations and demands encountered in the legal arena carry an elevated risk of ethical, regulatory, and malpractice complaints.

While it is commonplace for mental health professionals to have a role in the legal system, many training programs are lax in preparing trainees for forensic services. There is an appalling dearth of graduate-level courses to equip trainees for performing in forensic cases with competence and relative safety from complaints. More often than not, the practitioner will have to remedy this deficiency by individual, postgraduate effort.

Today's mental health practitioner has an irrefutable duty to contribute to the legal system, particularly through being available for expert testimony. Fulfilling this duty is part of the price tag for having the privilege of being deemed a professional by society.

This chapter covers numerous fundamentals for engaging in forensic services. Special attention will be given to being a fact and/or expert witness, managing forensic operations, receiving compensation, and accommodating clinical and other standards.

I am scheduled to appear as a witness in a case involving an ex-client. I called the attorney and stated that my expert fee was a certain amount, but was told that it would not be paid because I was being called as a "fact" witness. What is the difference between a "fact" witness and an "expert" witness?

If a person is witness to an event, he or she is potentially subject to be called to testify in a legal proceeding as a fact witness. A fact witness must testify about what was observed.

If a therapist serves as a fact witness, testimony about factual events will be required, such as verifying that the particular party in the legal action was provided with professional services, the dates and place for the services, the fees paid, and the records that were created. Production of the records will include the therapist's testimony that they are complete, true, and accurate.

An expert witness has the sole purpose of providing the trier of fact (the judge and/or the jury) with information derived from professional training and experience. With the therapist, it will involve providing information from behavioral science and professional experiences, presented in the form of opinions.

An expert opinion requires academic or scholarly underpinnings, coming from training and/or experience. Thus, questions for expert testimony might be about definition of clinical terms,

explanation of a diagnosis, justification for a treatment recommendation, or opinion about how mental health issues relate to
a particular legal issue.

As will be discussed in other questions and answers, a therapist can serve as either or both a fact witness and/or expert witness. The specific realm in which the therapist is to testify should
be determined, preferably at the first inkling of involvement in
the legal proceedings.

If the testimony is to be "fact" in nature, each jurisdiction
will have an established fee, which is typically quite nominal. If
the testimony is to be "expert" in nature, the therapist is entitled
to receive his or her professional fee. Unfortunately, some attorneys are prone to try to avoid paying the professional fee, yet
want to extract the expert opinions for the nominal fact witness
fee. Therefore, the therapist should address this matter early on.
Subsequent questions and answers clarify related issues.

**I received a subpoena from an attorney representing someone
who is suing an ex-client of mine. It was accompanied by a check
for $15, yet it required my showing up in court during a work-
day—this means I will lose a considerable amount of income. Do
I have to show up?**

Recall the preceding distinction made for the "fact" witness versus the "expert" witness. Given the amount of money sent, it
would appear that the subpoena is for fact testimony. In that case,
the therapist must appear, but only to give fact testimony.

Quite often, attorneys will attempt to transform a therapist's
appearance as a fact witness into being an expert witness. Commonly this transformation is motivated by a wish to avoid a professional fee, yet capitalize on the expertise of the therapist. The
attorney issuing the fact witness subpoena and payment has no
intention or willingness to pay a professional fee beyond the nominal fact witness fee.

Whenever a fact witness subpoena and fee are received, the
therapist should immediately send a letter (preferably by certified
mail), indicating that he or she will, of course, appear as a fact
witness, but assert that there will be no expert opinions rendered

unless there is a clear-cut written agreement that establishes the payment of a professional fee. Further, if the therapist is in a deposition when the transformation is attempted, he or she should respectfully decline to respond to opinion questions, that is, any question that relies upon the therapist's professional training as opposed to having simply been present when a factual event occurred (e.g., "Would you please define the clinical term in your report?").

The therapist must be prepared to stand firm and not be bullied or coerced into involuntarily becoming an expert witness. Again, it is possible to assert that, "I respectfully decline to answer, and request that you certify the question to the court as to whether or not I must serve as an expert witness without payment of my professional fee." If the attorney agrees to certify or submit the issue of a professional fee to the court, the therapist should reflect support of the judicial system by going ahead and answering opinion questions, even though the matter of being paid a professional fee remains unanswered.

Likewise, if the transformation is attempted while the therapist is in the courtroom, the therapist should request a ruling from the judge about whether or not expert testimony is required and, if so, how payment is to be made. If the professional fee is reasonable and proper deference to the court has been shown by the therapist, experience supports that judges will commonly order (or at least mediate) a payment arrangement.

Can I refuse to testify in a case involving one of my clients?

If subpoenaed to testify, the therapist is obligated to determine whether or not the subpoena has to be honored and, if so, to what extent. There seems little doubt that a therapist could be required to testify about any client he or she has treated. That is, any person is potentially subject to be subpoenaed to testify as to facts that are relevant and material to legal issues.

A therapist is not absolutely required to appear to testify as an expert. While issues of this nature are always subject to review by a court, there is good reason for believing that a therapist could establish, such as by the initial service contract, that he or she would or would not be available to serve as an expert witness in any legal action that involves the client, unless required by the court to do so. If there is willingness to potentially serve as an expert witness, before the fact there should be a written understanding about, among other things, the fee and payment arrangements. Of course, a service contract could not preclude the therapist's being called as a fact witness.

Since I dislike appearing in court, could I have each client sign an agreement before the first treatment session that would exempt me from ever having to appear in court?

See the preceding answer, but let us take the matter further. Within the mental health professions, there seems to be increasing concern about a possibly inappropriate dual relationship and/or conflict of interest for a therapist who provides both treatment and expert testimony. Some state regulatory agencies (e.g., via licensing boards) are promulgating rules on this matter, such as declaring that a therapist treating a child cannot also do a custody evaluation. Certain professional associations are also addressing this matter in their codes of ethics. To date, there is no clear-cut or universal legal position on a therapist's doing both treatment and expert testimony. The unique views or laws of the jurisdiction in which the therapist practices must be considered.

The question raises the possibility of the client's agreeing contractually not to ask the therapist to appear in court. Most basically, any contract must be conscionable in the eyes of the law. Since public policy endows the therapist with the privilege to practice and hold professional status, there is a distinct possibility that a court would view with disfavor any attempt by a therapist to avoid serving the judicial system if necessary. In other words, a client contract that agreed not to ask the therapist to appear in court would run the risk of being void by public policy or unconscionable in the mind of the court.

Further, simply because the client signs a contract not to ask the therapist to appear in court would not preclude a subpoena to testify coming from some other source. If the client becomes a party to a lawsuit, it seems certain that the opposing party would

consider whether or not the therapist's testimony would be helpful, and if properly subpoenaed, the therapist would be required
to appear and offer good faith fact testimony.

Could the opposing party require the therapist to give expert
testimony? Quite possibly, but this would be a matter for the court
to decide. If the answer were in the affirmative, the therapist
would have a legitimate claim to predicate his or her expert testimony on payment of the established professional fee.

**If I am giving expert testimony and a question is asked about
something that the client said that I should not tell anyone under
any circumstances, does professional privilege allow me to refuse
to answer the question or to deny knowing something that, in
fact, I do know?**

No one can lie under oath, and a therapist is no exception. Thus,
knowledge cannot be denied per se. If there is a question involving information that the client has refused to authorize the therapist to release or even discuss in general terms, the therapist can
properly and respectfully decline to answer, indicating the reason
for the refusal.

If this situation occurs in a deposition and the client's attorney or the client will not authorize a response and the opposing
counsel demands an answer, the therapist should politely but
firmly persist in refusing to answer and say (what the client's
attorney should have said by this point), "I respectfully object to
answering on behalf of my client's claim of confidentiality and
request that the question be certified to the court." Certifying a
question to the court means that the judge will decide whether
or not the therapist must answer a particular question, notwithstanding the client's claim to confidentiality. Some jurisdictions,
however, require that a question certified to the court be answered anyway, with the court's ruling determining whether it
will be admissible or inadmissible as evidence.

If this situation occurs in the courtroom, again the therapist
should respectfully decline to answer, explain the reason, and
wait for the judge to indicate whether or not the therapist should
answer the question. As always, if the court orders a response, it
should be given in unreserved fashion.

If I am in a deposition and I am not sure that I know the answer to a question, or it is something I do not believe I should answer, how do I appropriately avoid being forced into answering?

The previous question and answer indicates how to respond to a question that the therapist believes should not be answered, namely by certifying it to the court. The prudent therapist errs on the side of being overly cautious about answering questions, especially if there is any doubt as to the client's authorization to reveal confidential information.

If a question requires an answer that is outside the competency, training, or knowledge of the therapist, there should be no reluctance to admit readily, "I respectfully decline to answer that question because it is outside my area of expertise." Relatedly, questions often ask for an expert opinion with a "reasonable degree of professional certainty." The prudent therapist should never render an expert opinion, regardless of the degree of certainty, without a well-established academic rationale. Further, the academic rationale must be understood and capable of being expressed in a scholarly manner by the therapist.

Keep in mind that expert opinion is not personal opinion, it is a viewpoint predicated on behavioral science, academic, or scholarly information and research. On the latter factor, if a particular question asks for an answer that cannot be formulated without a body of research and there is no such corpus of scientific or scholarly information, the therapist should decline to answer.

There is no reason for a therapist to be tentative about admitting to his or her limits of competency. To the contrary, there are numerous ethical and legal reasons why there must never be a response by a therapist that is presented as being "professional" unless the therapist has adequate training and knowledge to the degree expected for the prevailing minimum standards of the relevant profession.

Too often, a therapist tries to bluff his or her way through a response, thinking erroneously that this will benefit the client. In point of fact, it stands to be potentially detrimental to the client, especially if the therapist's credibility is impeached (e.g., during cross-examination).

Some therapists present testimony without adequate or documentable expertise because of inadvertence or a momentary delusion of grandeur. This faux pas may occur because of an illogical (perhaps unconscious) wish to further the legal benefits for the client, or it may be due to a narcissistic (perhaps unconscious) motive to appear to be an esteemed expert. Such a temptation must be rejected—to succumb to it will lead to negative consequences.

I received a subpoena today about noon, stating that I have to be in court tomorrow at 9:00 A.M. "or any time thereafter indicated by the court." I telephoned the attorney who sent the subpoena. In a gruff voice, I was told that I had to be there, with an "or else you will suffer the consequences" tone. It will mean canceling a full day of clients who are scheduled for sessions. Seems like the attorney could have given me some advance notice, then I would certainly cooperate. What are my options?

Assuming that the subpoena is for fact testimony, it would be quite proper for the therapist to immediately enter an objection and motion to the court, indicating that his or her legal duties to other previously scheduled clients would potentially have to be violated by honoring a subpoena that does not specify a specific date and time. While there may be variation, most courts are prone to support a bona fide professional concern about the welfare of other clients; and it seems likely, all things being equal, that the court would arrange for the attorneys to have the therapist present according to a fixed schedule, even if it meant interrupting other testimony that was in process or scheduled.

Oftentimes, the therapist's objection to an ambiguous appearance subpoena is more a matter of money than avoiding infringement on the rights of other clients. That is, the therapist is concerned about having considerable "down time" while waiting to appear. If avoiding loss of income is the motive, being a fact witness will not accommodate a more specific schedule. It is like jury duty—there comes a time when everyone must serve. If the therapist has voluntarily entered into the role of expert witness, there should be an established contractual arrangement for payment that would assure the therapist of compensation for all time (or lost income), including "down time" while waiting to be called to testify. If there is no such agreement, the therapist has only him- or herself to blame.

If I get a subpoena from another state, do I have to travel there to give testimony?

It all depends on why the therapist was selected to receive the subpoena and what the laws are for the issuing jurisdiction. Assuming that there was jurisdiction over the therapist, a therapist who is a party to legal action potentially may be reached in another state by the "long arm" statute of the jurisdiction in which the case is filed.

There have been instances involving a therapist who provided treatment to a client in State A, the client moved to State B, and became a party to a legal action, and the client's attorney attempted to subpoena the therapist from State A to appear in State B, usually for the purpose of expert testimony. In this situation, it is unlikely that the jurisdiction for State B would justify subpoena power in State A. Nonetheless, upon receiving the subpoena the therapist should have an attorney file an objection with the court that issued the subpoena (or an order to appear). Of course the therapist could agree to appear in State B, but it would be illogical to do so unless the client had made payment for the professional services, preferably in advance.

Since there is typically some uncertainty about the authority of a subpoena issued from another jurisdiction, it is always wise to turn this matter over to an attorney to handle in formal fashion. While the therapist may incur some expense for legal representation, this is a necessary business expense in the present-day litigious era.

Even though I never had any contact with either of them, a divorcing couple told a judge that they wanted me to do an evaluation of their children for custody and visitation matters. Through the mail, I received a legal document titled "Order," and in it the judge states that I shall do the evaluation. I am overloaded already. Do I have to do this case because the judge said so?

Generally, a therapist does not have to accept any case, but if an order involving the therapist is issued, in deference to the court the therapist must be responsive. Being overloaded, with preexisting duties to other clients, is usually an adequate reason to have the order rescinded. There is little or no legal justification for placing would-be clients' rights above the rights of established clients.

Usually there is no reason to be upset or cantankerous about this sort of situation. It is almost always sufficient to simply inform the court of the undue hardship that would be created (such as for meeting the established legal duties to other clients) or a personal wish of the therapist to not be involved. More often than not, the court was acting on a recommendation from an attorney, who thought that the particular therapist would be most useful to his or her client's interests, and was not aware that the therapist might object to being involved in the case. To avoid any misstep, it would probably be best for the therapist to have an attorney take care of this matter.

I received a court order indicating that I should provide counseling to the children and parents in a divorcing family. When I called the parents, who are now living apart, each of them said basically the same thing, "I'll come to see you because the judge ordered it, but I can't afford to pay anything—talk to my *#!@ spouse about paying." Who is going to pay for my services?

If the parties cannot afford to pay the therapist's professional fee, it is potentially wrongful for a court to order the therapist to provide services for no payment. Under laws of the particular jurisdiction, the court might have discretion in fixing the fee, but under federal law, notably the U.S. Constitution, there cannot be an unlawful taking of property by the government. It would seem that governmental ordering of services for inadequate or no compensation is potentially an unlawful taking of personal property (i.e., the therapist's professional expertise constitutes intellectual property), as well as a possible violation of other rights.

Before scheduling an appointment to see a court-ordered client, provisions should be made for payment. In the event that an acceptable payment arrangement is not agreed upon, the therapist should (preferably through his or her legal counsel) submit a motion to the court asking to be dismissed from the case. Since the good will of the court must be maintained, and it must be treated with respect, care should be exercised to be tactful. Thus, this is another situation for which it would be advisable for the therapist to have an attorney take care of the matter.

5

Dual Relationships

The nature of the therapeutic relationship has been, as it should be, in a constant state of evolution. Concurrently, public policy and the law have also changed in ways that affect the relationship between the therapist and client.

Psychotherapy achieved its most rapid and substantial advances from the 1950s through the 1970s. While there was a plethora of therapeutic theories, there seemed to be an omnipresent humanistic component, which tended to oppose the therapist's being more "powerful" than the client. Consequently, a therapist was encouraged to set aside professional status and deal with a client as a peer. As might be expected, this approach opened up the possibility of conduct that contradicted professionalism. In some instances, these unrestrained therapeutic relationships reflected more a quest for need fulfillment for the therapist than benefits for the client.

In the late 1960s and early 1970s, the so-called human potential movement epitomized the exploration of unique therapist and client contacts. The client's psychological growth was thought to be facilitated by the therapist's fostering intense encounters and unguarded interactions, which extended to highly personalized sharing of minds and bodies by the therapist and client.

Often, this exchange resulted in multiple roles, such as the therapist and client expanding their "treatment" relationship to education, business, social, romantic, and sexual interactions.

Given the evolution of public attitudes toward health care in general and mental health in particular, today most of society emphatically rejects almost all multiple relationships between the therapist and client. While feasibly there are some "dual" relationships that would be acceptable under unique circumstances, the trend is to view any therapeutic relationship that includes dual purposes as suspect and potentially unacceptable.

If a dual relationship is condemned or proscribed by public policy or law, the sanctions can be profound. For example, most jurisdictions hold that any sexual encounter between a therapist and a client is subject to legal action. Some jurisdictions criminalize such sexual contacts and/or prohibit sexual relations between the therapist and client in perpetuity.

The potential for liability from dual relationships continues to be extended further. Even if the client condones a unique relationship, a therapist who interacts with a client beyond a conservative role definition is vulnerable to censure.

This chapter explores a variety of situations that might have been acceptable in another era, but today must be either avoided or carefully controlled. The outcome will be a risk management plan by which the prudent practitioner can construct therapeutic relationships that will be both helpful to the client and legally safe for the practitioner.

I live in a small town, and through my church, children's school, and other community activities, I know just about everyone, indirectly if not directly. I would like to set up a private practice, but I am worried about having almost all of my potential clients being people with whom I have some other sort of preexisting relationship. Is the bottom line that I have to stay out of practice?

Trying to live and practice in a small town carries more likelihood of problematic contacts than would be likely to occur in a large city. A therapist need not stay out of practice, but certain steps should be taken to minimize the possibility of inappropriate dual relationships.

In a nutshell, the mental health practitioner in a small town should avoid providing extensive services to folks with whom there have been personal contacts or relations, including their immediate family members. Instead of psychotherapy, the focus should be on supportive and information-giving services, with the goal to motivate the person(s) to seek services elsewhere.

The fact that the practice is in a small town does not exempt the practitioner from the ethical and legal pitfalls associated with inappropriate dual relationships and the concomitants of conflict of interests and undue influence. The risk will exist, and there is no safe solution except to serve as a referral source when a dual relationship is apparent.

I get referrals for child custody evaluations from a prominent domestic lawyer. She has just called me and wants me to start treating her teenage daughter. My concern is twofold. If I treat her daughter, something negative about the mother or family might emerge or the daughter may end up going in a direction that disappoints her mother, and I might be blamed. If I refuse to treat her daughter, the mother might stop referring custody evaluation cases to me. I hate to lose her referrals, but it looks like I am destined, as the adage says, to be "damned if I do and damned if I don't."

The adage cited does apply. Having developed confidence in the therapist's ability, entrusting the welfare of the teenager is understandable. Nonetheless, there is liability associated with accepting this sort of dual relationship. As a rule of thumb, when the therapist has extensive contacts in one role with a person, it is potentially inappropriate to move to another role, even with the person's approval.

Certainly it is desirable to retain the attorney's acceptance for continuing referrals for child custody evaluations. With this scenario, it would be prudent for the therapist to keep the intervention at a supportive and information-giving level, and promote referral to another treatment source. This referral strategy should be framed as maximizing the benefits for the teenager. In turn, it will possibly strengthen the relationship with the attorney for future referrals for child custody evaluations.

I work for a clinic as a therapist and also serve on a board for a community nonprofit agency for youth. To my horror, the agency is seriously considering the possibility of hiring a former patient who, maybe a decade ago, was diagnosed as a pedophile. He was not my patient, but I heard all about his diagnosis and treatment in our staff conferences and remember the sordid details. So far I have said nothing to the agency, but I really fear that if he is hired, his access to the youth in the program will be potentially problematic for all concerned, including the former patient. I talked to the director of our clinic, and was told that I am duty bound to maintain confidentiality and if I say anything to the agency, I will be fired. If the agency hires this man and abuse occurs, I gather I might have legal liability. How on earth do I get out of this mess?

The previously cited adage, "Damned if I do, and damned if I don't" finds ready application again. The client diagnosed as a pedophile does have a right to maintenance of privileged communications. While jurisdictions vary in definition of the "duty to warn," breaching confidentiality on the basis of protecting others usually requires that the danger of violence or bodily harm be imminent. With the scenario set forth in this question, it is known that about a decade has passed since the diagnosis and there is no known immediate danger. At the most, there seems to be only a possibility of danger, which is based on old information.

Nonetheless, the therapist has a distinct legal risk. If the therapist does not act upon the knowledge of past treatment and (even tacitly) goes along with the hiring of the patient, and then the patient does abuse a youth and it emerges that the therapist had the knowledge of past pedophilia, it is quite likely that legal action against the therapist would be possible.

"Getting out of this mess" is not easily accomplished. The most logical first step would be to tactfully request that the patient return to the clinic for a session, wherein the dilemma would be presented. If the patient could not or would not provide current information sufficient to reasonably assuage concerns about the potential for abuse of youths or refused to withdraw his application for the employment, the therapist would have little option but to immediately withdraw from the deliberations of the community nonprofit agency for youth. If the latter action is taken, the therapist could not provide a reason, other than something along the lines of "inappropriate dual relations" or "conflict of interests." Even then, the legal risk continues.

I agree that therapists should not have sex with their clients. However, I am single and have had a number of clients who would be nice to date. If I terminate therapy, how long do I have to wait before I can date a former client?

In their codes of ethics, certain professional associations have included time frames for when a social or sexual relationship between a therapist and a past client is no longer unethical. From the legal point of view, such a time frame is illogical.

Under law, a statute of limitation (which varies among jurisdictions) commonly accommodates a legal action against a therapist beyond the time frames that are found in the codes of ethics. A time frame in a code of ethics would not, of course, negate legal prescriptions and proscriptions.

There is considerable variation between state statutes on the issues related to a therapist and client having social or sexual relations, and common or case law rulings are even more diverse. Some jurisdictions allow criminal, regulatory, and civil (e.g., malpractice) actions against a therapist who engages in a sexual relationship with a client, even if the former client voluntarily entered into the relationship. Some jurisdictions include in their licensing laws that for purposes of sexual misconduct, the relationship between a therapist and client is deemed to be in perpetuity (i.e., forever).

The foregoing means that there is no time frame for a social or sexual relationship with a former client. There are many legal cases that occurred when a former patient ended a romantic relationship with a therapist. Despite the patient's voluntary entry into the relationship after therapy had been concluded, he or she alleges that but for the unequal power or undue influence accorded to the therapist by the past professional relationship, the relationship would not have occurred and the patient was, therefore, damaged.

While perhaps difficult to accept, the prudent ethical and legal view should be: Once a client, always a client. At the risk of seeming impolite, if a therapist cannot find social or romantic companions from other than a pool of persons to whom the therapist has provided treatment, perhaps he or she should seek professional help.

Once after a session, I stopped in a restaurant-bar in the same shopping plaza as my office, and encountered a client. We sat at the bar and had a few drinks. Now it has sort of become a regular event: The client has a session with me, usually at the end of the day, leaves, and I go to the bar knowing full well that the client will be there. We are both single. So far we have just had these friendly discussions, and there does not seem to be any adverse effects in therapy. Is this acceptable professionally?

This situation is wrong professionally and reflects poorly on the professional and personal qualities of the therapist. The legal risks are multiple and extreme. There is no logical justification. As for not having any adverse effects in therapy, it seems improbable that the therapist can objectively assess the effects. From the mental health practice and legal risk management points of view, both the therapeutic and the social relationships should be terminated immediately, with a proper referral of the client to another practitioner. Given the substance of the question, it seems clear that the therapist likely needs professional help, be it for supervision of practice or personal problems.

More than a decade ago when I was a professor, I had a student with whom I had several counseling sessions, just dealing with educational plans. A few months ago we bumped into each other at a professional meeting. We are both mental health practitioners, have been dating, and plan to be married. Why do I have this gnawing doubt about the propriety of this involvement with a past student-counselee?

Recall the previous question and answer about a waiting period for socializing with a former client, and the recommendation that the prudent stance is "once a client, always a client." The nature of the earlier intervention (i.e., educational planning) and the lengthy passage of time without contacts (i.e., more than a decade) seem to minimize the possibility of allegations of impropriety. Regardless, there is a dual relationship that is interwoven into the fabric of the relationship. It remains for conjecture how, if at all, this dual relationship will impact on future marital relations.

I married one of my patients. Do I have any legal risk?

In principle, there is always a risk that an inappropriate dual relationship will carry the risk of legal action. While sanctified by law and religion, marrying a client is not immune from the possibility of negative allegations. If the marriage turns sour, the former client may recast what seemed like a straightforward courtship as having been enticement, solicitation, harassment, or undue influence or control that was only possible because of the therapist's power.

In some jurisdictions, the "in perpetuity concept" keeps open the possibility of numerous sources, such as competitive therapists in the community, submitting a complaint to an ethics committee or a regulatory agency. To have a complaint, there must be a complainant.

When discussing an upcoming marriage of a psychologist to one of her former client's, a member of a state licensing board commented, "She had better keep him happy!" Sure enough, only a few months after the marriage, she decided to seek a divorce, and her husband filed a complaint against her. Beyond alleging undue influence, he pointed out that the psychologist had testified as an expert in his custody proceedings, and started dating him only a short time thereafter.

Stated bluntly, marriage does not absolve the therapist of liability.

I have a client who is unemployed and has trouble paying for treatment. I could use the client as an office worker on a part-time basis. I have an office manager who would be the direct supervisor. Is this enough distance between me and the client?

This employment arrangement does not afford enough distance between the therapist and the client. In one such instance, the employee-client proved incompetent, and the employer, her therapist, had to terminate her employment. Since she had sought treatment for poor self-esteem and her therapist-employer had validated her incompetence, the negative impact was severe.

There is no way to justify a dual relationship that carries the potential of inflicting injury on a client. While a client may need employment, the appropriate strategy would be to provide career counseling, not employment.

One of my past clients has contacted me about a possible business investment. I saw him for only a few sessions. He was a well-adjusted fellow who just wanted some help sharpening his career goals. In the meantime, he has done very well and is presenting me with a chance to invest money in a project that will likely produce financial benefits. I would not be involved in managerial decision making; I would just invest the money as a so-called "limited partner." Do I have any possible professional conflict?

By contemporary professional standards, any dual relationship involving a therapist and a client is subject to being wrongful or inappropriate. While the client may be well adjusted and seemingly strong psychologically, there is still the potential for an allegation of unequal power in the relationship.

In one such situation, the therapist made a substantial investment of money and remained a passive partner. When the business succeeded, an attorney for the client contacted the therapist with an offer to refund exactly the same amount of money that the therapist had invested. The therapist expressed the belief that he or she should receive more than the initial investment because of the success of the venture. The client's attorney responded that unless the refund was accepted, a legal complaint would be filed alleging that the therapist had, among other possible breaches of the standards for the profession, exercised undue influence in getting the client to accept the investment. After accepting the refund, the therapist ruefully commented that, ''I suppose that if the business had failed, I would have been liable for the investment made by the client as well.''

I have clients who provide services, like carpentry, or who have

property, like a motorcycle, that I would be willing to accept instead of money. If we can agree on the value of the services or property, can we make the swap?

Because of the assumed unequal bargaining power between a therapist and client, codes of ethics tend to caution against or actually proscribe bartering. That is, bartering is viewed as being a high risk for unethical conduct and should be avoided. Whenever a therapist acts counter to what might be the prevailing standard for the profession, there is legal risk. The answer is simple: "Do not barter, there is too much risk associated with it."

My spouse and I are remodeling our home. After receiving several bids, it is clear that the best offer comes, as fate would have it, from an ex-client of mine. I have not seen the person for about five years. Is it all right to let the ex-client do the work?

As exemplified in previous questions and answers, there may be legal risks associated with doing business with a former client. For example, what if the client does the project for X-amount and later wants additional payment, alleging that the X-amount would not have been agreed to but for the therapist's special power.

Keep in mind that even a contract can be found to be unconscionable because of undue influence, mental incompetency, distress, or other conditions that might be associated with the therapist–client relationship. Further, the negative view about dual relationships held by public policy and legal sources would likely mean that the presumption of wrongdoing would remain for the therapist to counter, as opposed to the presumption that the client made an informed decision.

My spouse has a service business. One of my clients is in need of that kind of service. Can I recommend that the client contact my spouse?

It is ill advised to make any recommendation that is beyond the perimeter of treatment or that benefits the therapist beyond the customary fee. Soliciting business for a spouse or any other source would not be therapeutic, and it would be impossible to justify the propriety of such a recommendation to the client.

As a rule of thumb, it is best not to do anything that was not taught in a professional training program or for which there is no behavioral science research or legal authority. Instead of adopting the view that, "If it is not prohibited, I can do it," the prudent therapist maintains, "If it is not authorized professionally, I will not do it."

A couple who are both therapists here in town have really enjoyable parties. I have noticed, however, that some of the folks attending the parties are former clients of the hosts. When I tactfully asked them about the wisdom of inviting clients, they joked about it, saying that "they have graduated from therapy, they can't remain clients forever." Am I foolish to feel squeamish about seeing former clients at the therapists' parties?

It is not foolish to avoid giving explicit or implicit support to any therapist's conduct that may be inappropriate. By condoning another therapist's social relations with clients, there is an acceptance of responsibility. Socializing with clients, past or present, is a disservice to the client's therapeutic benefits and to the status of the profession.

Several of my clients have given me personal gifts, like books, jewelry, and odds and ends for my office. One client, who is also a mental health professional, has been giving me more expensive items. Every time I resist the gift, the client gets aggravated, almost hostile, and forces me to keep the gift. What do I do?

All gifts should be avoided because gift giving redefines the relationship. The relationship is predicated upon exchange theory, but with terms and considerations (e.g., the professional fee) recognized by the discipline and society.

Small items of no significant financial value (say a greeting card or homemade candy) would be less risky than more expensive items, but they will convey a negative message about the quality of the professional relationship.

There have been many legal complaints against therapists that include allegations that the therapist should not have accepted gifts, even though the clients insisted on it at the time.

For example, one client insisted that the therapist accept numerous gifts. Later, when the therapist tried to collect an overdue account, the client filed a regulatory complaint and a malpractice action, alleging that the therapist had accepted all sorts of gifts (e.g., handkerchiefs, books about self-growth and poetry, flowers, candy, rare coins, etc.). Fortunately, the therapist had wisely kept and cataloged all of the items and had his attorney return them to the plaintiff's attorney immediately, along with an affidavit that the gifts were never solicited or wanted, and were held in escrow for the client.

A client left a bicycle in front of my office. The client is a wanderer and has not been seen or heard from since, and I have no known address. I have kept the bike for several months. I do not have a place for it and would like to get rid of it. How do I go about it?

While there are more formal methods, such as giving constructive notice by running an announcement in a newspaper, it would seem that there is not much that can be done with what amounts to abandoned property. Certainly the therapist should make a note for the client's record, indicating that the item was left, the fact that there was no known address, and the length of time that it was retained—then disposal of the bicycle would probably be in order. Instead of keeping it for personal use or selling it, it would be better to give it to a charitable organization. In principle, if the client shows up later wanting the bicycle, the prudent action would be to buy another one for the client without any ado.

6

Records

Records constitute one of the most critical aspects of professional mental health services. Thoughtful and detailed recording of what has transpired in a professional relationship can benefit the client if he or she seeks other professional services later on. Of equal importance (albeit often foolishly minimized or overlooked) is the benefit to the practitioner, namely documentation of treatment as relevant to standard of care, risk management, and legal liability.

Inexplicably, some mental health practitioners harbor a notion that records are unnecessary. Their reasoning is often along these lines, "If I am writing notes in the presence of the client, he or she will be more guarded in what will be revealed," or "Writing notes after a session is too time consuming and I will forget important information." Another rationalization is, "If the client tells me something detrimental to his or her interests and I write it down, the client could be damaged in any legal action that occurs later on."

None of the foregoing notions has credibility. The practitioner is obligated to record and retain information about the client, whether the notes are made during or after the session in which the information was transmitted. Also, it is not for the practitioner to be concerned about what the information is used for later on, as long as it is properly released. For example, in a legal action, advocacy to keep potentially detrimental information out of legal proceedings is the responsibility, indeed the duty, of the client's attorney, not the therapist.

As a result of faulty record keeping by mental health practitioners, some jurisdictions have promulgated statutes and/or rules that mandate the making and retention of records, and specify conditions for the content, storage, and release of records. Professional associations have followed this course of action by upgrading their ethics relevant to records.

This chapter will provide a detailed accounting of what ethics and laws expect of the mental health practitioner when it comes to records. It is axiomatic that there must be comprehensive records, and safeguards for storage and release of records.

What should be contained in a client's clinical record?

The two primary purposes for making and keeping records should be recognized. First, the records document what services were provided and information needed to familiarize all subsequent health care professionals with what did or did not help the client. Second, the records document the quality of care provided to the client, thereby serving an important risk management purpose for the benefit of the therapist.

As for what should be entered into the records, the determination must be made according to what is required by the laws of the jurisdiction, the treatment needs of the client, and the risk management system of the therapist. The trend seems to be for state licensing laws and their concomitant rules to prescribe what should be the minimal contents of the treatment record, as well as how the records should be retained (e.g., length of retention). Certain professional associations also cover these matters in their codes of ethics, but of course ethics do not supersede laws.

Statutory and common laws, ethics, and prevailing standards for the mental health disciplines support basing all therapy on an individualized treatment plan. In this day and age of managed health care, accountability mandates a detailed and monitored treatment plan.

For risk management, it is essential to make as many entries of what the therapist says and does as of what the client says and does. Keep in mind that legal actions are, for the most part, based on what the therapist does or does not do, rather than on the client's conduct.

How long should I retain client records?

There is no one answer. Ethical rules within the discipline and laws for the jurisdiction must be considered. Legal considerations support keeping the records for many years, perhaps forever.

I figure the less said in session notes the better, right?

Nothing could be more wrong—the more details, the better. This assumes, of course, that the contents of the records are substantive and aligned with the two primary purposes set forth earlier (i.e., quality care for the client and risk management for the therapist). Carefully made and comprehensive records will benefit both client and therapist. Courts tend to give deference to records that are made contemporaneously. It is reasoned that if the comments were written into the records immediately upon or after the treatment session, the substance is valid and honest.

I work for a family social agency that has a policy that therapists should keep no case notes. This seems wrong to me. What should I do?

An agency policy does not supersede the law. Care must be taken to keep records that are in accord with the laws of the jurisdiction(s). Moreover, as stated earlier, records are kept for the future treatment benefit of the client and for the risk management benefit of the therapist.

When a therapist works for an agency that has an unethical, illogical, or illegal policy about records, the therapist should assertively educate the administration to the essential and/or mandatory reasons for changing the policy. At some juncture, it may come to be that the therapist will be forced to choose between either continuing to work under the unprofessional, illegal, or risky conditions, or terminating employment and seeking more professional, legal, and safe employment elsewhere.

It seems that, more often than not, when an agency has an illogical or illegal policy, it is merely the tip of the legal-risk iceberg. When a legal disaster strikes, it is a safe bet that the agency will not back the therapist, and the therapist's personal reputation and resources will potentially be subject to a punitive outcome.

Stated bluntly, if the therapist cannot quickly and promptly accomplish a remedy with an errant agency, it is foolhardy to continue to be employed there. In the long run, no matter what reassurances are given by the employer, they are unlikely to provide the professional, legal, and financial safeguards that are necessary for protecting the therapist.

One of my associates is leaving my employment, and says that state law requires the therapist to keep and maintain records. Since the therapist worked for me, I am aware that I have liability for his or her clients and may need those records myself. I do not want to risk having those records disappear or not be available to me. Also, I have a hunch that the therapist would use those records to solicit the clients to her new practice, which would be taking away part of my new practice. What are my rights?

Certain states do have laws, usually under licensing statutes or rules, that prescribe that a licensed therapist is required to make and retain records. While a particular jurisdiction may be different, most often the wording is intended to assure that the client can, if ever needed, obtain the records, as opposed to declaring that the therapist who provided the service has a superior claim over the employer for ownership of the records.

The records made by employees are considered to be "property," for which the employer would generally have ownership property rights. Indeed, state laws commonly identify the business records (which would include clinical records) of an employer as potentially containing "trade secrets" and being entitled to special protections from use by others. Therefore, when an employee departs and tries to make use of lists of client addresses, the employer can seek an injunction to prohibit the employee from having information, possession of which would result in unfair competition with the employer's business (other remedies are usually also available to the employer).

Aside from future business per se, the employer does have liability for the conduct of employees, and the records are critically important for any legal matter that might eventuate under the *respondeat superior* or master–servant principles. The possible conflict between an employee–therapist's duty to retain records and the ownership rights of the employer is often addressed by regulatory agencies. While not fully settled, it appears that the trend is toward allowing priority to the employer's rights, as long as the employer abides by relevant retention laws and agrees to retain the records and make them available to the clients and treating therapist as may be necessary for future clinical or legal purposes. Certainly both the employer and the employee should be assured that the records will be retained and accessible when justified.

Virtually every day, I return calls from clients from my home, and commonly get involved in rather substantive conversations. Should I be taking notes on these conversations and making them part of clients' clinical files?

Yes, notes should be kept of every communication with or about a client, regardless of context or source. The notion is that but for the professional relationship, the therapist would not be communicating with or about the client. Therefore, the communication should be retained as part of the clinical records, for the purposes discussed previously.

There have been innumerable legal claims against therapists based on communications that allegedly occurred outside of the treatment room or were not included in the clinical records. In many of these instances, the deference to contemporaneously made notes that would be granted by the court would have paved the way to effectively countering the allegations, but only if there were, in fact, contemporaneously made notes that were preserved in the clinical record.

A good method is to have a prepared form (rather than a scrap of paper) next to the telephone at home, which would allow a uniform and systematic record of every telephone conversation with or about a client. If the communication should occur elsewhere (e.g., returning a "call back" message from a client while the therapist is, say, at a restaurant), a written record should be made (on the standard form) as soon as the therapist returns to the office.

I prefer to keep two sets of notes, one that I consider to be the client's clinical records and one that I consider to be my "personal notes" about my treatment of the client. Is it possible that I could be forced to reveal my "personal notes" to the client?

Absolutely yes, any record that is subpoenaed is potentially subject to discovery or legally mandated production, regardless of any self-ordained "for my use only" status. If all records are not produced in response to a proper subpoena, the therapist will be vulnerable to all sorts of possible legal actions, not the least of which will be a motion for a contempt of court, along with, possibly, a complaint to the licensing agency alleging breach of the minimum standards for the profession.

Jurisdictions vary about what records a client can demand without a subpoena. While a jurisdiction might have a law that requires only "a summary of treatment" or a "clinical report," it is obvious that refusing to provide a client with any and all of his or her own clinical records is fraught with risk.

Given the purposes for keeping the records, there is typically no reason for not making records available to a client, with or without a subpoena. If there is a seemingly useful reason, such as clinical terminology that might not be in the best interest of the client, consideration should be given to counseling with the client about the reason; that is, face the issue directly and constructively, as opposed to being oppositional. Moreover, it should be pondered why the records, since they are for the benefit of the client, contain material that is inappropriate for the client to know.

If there is a strong, professional reason why certain records should not be released, again with or without a subpoena, the therapist is not endowed with the authority to solely determine the matter. Rather, when there is a dispute of any nature, and certainly a dispute over records between a therapist and a client is no exception, the prudent strategy is to put the matter to the court. For example, if records are subpoenaed by the client, a motion for a protective order can be filed for a judicial determination. It is feasible that, besides saying yes or no to releasing the records, the court might require releasing only certain parts of the records.

If a parent of a teenager who I am treating contacts me and wants a copy of the child's records and the teenager does not want the parent to see them, does the parent have a legal right to the records?

Generally speaking, children do not have certain legal rights; their legal rights are held by and exercised at the discretion of their parents or guardians. Thus, parents commonly have a right to copies of their children's health care records.

Some jurisdictions have laws or concomitant rules that hold that any person (regardless of age) receiving mental health services from a licensed practitioner has a right to have his or her communications treated as privileged information, which means parents would not definitely have a right to access the child's treatment records. Or conditions can be set whereby a therapist can potentially refuse to release records for the child, based on the therapist's conclusion that releasing the information would not be in the child's best interest (e.g., warring parents trying to manipulate therapeutic information in a custody dispute). Of course if the parents obtain a court order for production of the records, the records must be provided, notwithstanding the child's or therapist's preference to the contrary.

I resent health insurance companies wanting my clinical records for clients for whom they are making payments. Is there any way I can avoid turning over the records to them?

Cautious resistance to benefit the client might be appropriate, but any manifestation of one's personal opposition to insurance companies obtaining records is inadvisable. There may be a situation in which providing certain information to the insurance company would place the client at risk, say, of unemployment or other penalty; the therapist could appropriately, and with the client's approval, try to persuade the insurance carrier that only certain information is necessary for its purposes.

It must be recognized that the client agreed to certain contractual terms when accepting the policy coverage sold by the insurance company. Commonly one of the terms is that the client waive confidentiality relevant to providing any and all records requested by the insurance company. If the client entered properly into this contractual arrangement, it is not for the therapist to oppose it on personal principle.

One of my clients did not like her results on the MMPI-2, and demands that I tear up the answer sheet and protocol and remove all comments about the results from the clinical file. Do I have to destroy the test results?

No records, be they test results or otherwise, should ever be destroyed simply because any one person, be it client or therapist, does not like the contents. If the document contains information that is relevant and material to the clinical purposes of the client and/or the risk management purposes of the therapist, it should be retained.

Further, the therapist has a so-called "limited property right" in the document itself. If nothing else, the therapist paid for the paper and owns it. Therefore, no one but the therapist can require the destruction of a record without judicial order.

Some jurisdictions, by statutory or case law, hold that a destroyed or altered clinical record will be interpreted in the least favorable light for the record holder. This means that any relevant legal action would likely carry a presumption of wrongdoing on the part of the therapist (i.e., the record holder) that would have to be rebutted; and without the document, rebuttal would be difficult or impossible to accomplish.

Assume that a therapist honored a client's demand for destruction of an MMPI-2 protocol and the test data were needed later by the client. It would be quite appropriate for the client to take legal action against the therapist and allege that the destruction of the protocol was in violation of the best interests of the client and that, notwithstanding the client's request, the therapist should have refused to destroy the test—the clinical purpose of benefiting the client had not been served by the destruction. Or assume that the client later files a legal action against the therapist for, say, misdiagnosis, and the destroyed MMPI-2 protocol was the basis of support for the therapist's diagnosis—the risk management purpose to benefit the therapist would not be served by the destruction.

One of my clients is demanding that I "turn over" his file to him, saying that "it belongs" to him. Is the client right?

No, the client does not own or control possession of the document. The client only has a legal right that the information contained in the records be safeguarded. The client does not have the right to require the document to be destroyed, as long as the record containing the confidential information is being properly safeguarded. Recall that the therapist has a "limited property right" in the documents. The sole ownership of the records rests with the therapist.

I am treating a fellow who admits to murdering a fellow soldier during combat. It happened several years ago, and I do not believe anything would be gained by bringing it out now. The poor patient has enough problems already. Can I omit mention of this crime in the clinical record?

Omitting any relevant or material information that emerges in treatment, regardless of how negative for the client it may be, imposes a legal risk on the therapist. For example, what if this client commits a violent act, say, kills another person, and it emerges that he or she had told the therapist about the previous murder? To benefit the client, his or her attorney might well allege that such a violent previous act created a duty for the therapist to intervene in such a way as to prevent the client from committing future violence, and by failing to properly weigh that

information, the client suffered the negative consequences and
the therapist should be held liable:

> Ladies and gentlemen of the jury, the defendant-therapist did not
> even include mention of the previous murder in the clinical rec-
> ord, yet here in my client's diary are repeated entries indicating
> the therapist had been told about the violent acts that my client
> committed during combat—because of the defendant-therapist's
> failure to take adequate professional action to prevent additional
> violence, my client was tried for murder but found not guilty by
> reason of insanity, and has suffered and will suffer a lifetime of
> mental distress and other compensable damages because of the
> therapist's malpractice.

Keep in mind that the clinical record is for the benefit of
both client and therapist. While at first glance it might seem as
though omitting certain information will benefit the client, consideration must also be given to whether or not it will benefit
the therapist.

Further, the purpose of recordkeeping is to document the
services provided to the client. If the client possesses and commu-
nicates information that is relevant to the services provided, it
should be entered in the record. It is not for the therapist to
surreptitiously screen information to construct a record that will
protect the client from other possible monitors. To try to justify
this sort of judgment is to move far beyond society's endorsement
for mental health practitioners, and leaves the therapist exposed
to significant professional and legal risks.

**One of my clients is involved with selling drugs, and wants my
guarantee that I will not report him or her. Can I give such a guarantee?**

No, there can never be an unqualified guarantee that confidential
information will not be revealed. Virtually every state has statutes
that mandate reporting of certain types of information, such as
about child abuse.

While jurisdictions vary a bit, commonly a therapist does not
have to report criminal conduct (unless otherwise prescribed by

statute). Of course, certain conduct may trigger a duty to warn. Even though the nexus between selling drugs and violence may not be incontrovertible, it seems relatively easy to see that a therapist's knowledge of a client selling drugs could lead to possible violence or physical injury to self or others. Thus, depending on the circumstances, a "duty to warn" might develop. Further, there would also be the potential risk of the therapist allegedly aiding and abetting criminal activity.

Of greatest significance, however, is the fact that any information known to a therapist is potentially discoverable by legal process. Therefore, a properly implemented subpoena could lead to a legal mandate that the therapist reveal certain information that the client would rather have kept confidential. If the therapist had foolishly told the client that certain nefarious information, such as about drug sales, would not be revealed under any circumstances and legal process then required the revelation, the client, no matter how criminal his or her conduct, would potentially have a basis for legal action against the therapist.

From individual sessions with a couple to whom I am providing marital therapy, I know that each of them is quite promiscuous, but neither spouse knows about the other's sexual behavior. From my reading about affairs, I know that this is an issue that has implications for marital therapy; and in this age of sexually transmittable diseases, I am concerned about the risk promiscuity poses to the transgressor, as well as the unsuspecting spouse. What are the legal issues here?

Sexually transmittable diseases constitute a fairly new realm of concern for marriage therapy. Jurisdictions are just starting to formulate legal guidelines. While not indelibly written any place or universal in acceptance, there may be a trend emerging that grants immunity from legal action (such as for alleged breach of confidentiality) for a therapist's revealing to a spouse that the other spouse has acquired immune deficiency syndrome (AIDS). Whether this will extend to warning nonspouses who are at risk of infection remains for conjecture.

Also, there is a modicum of legal movement toward making it a crime for a person with AIDS to knowingly endanger a sexual partner. How this movement progresses, such as whether there will be criminalization of negligent exposure of partners to sexually transmittable diseases (only AIDS or other STDs as well?) remains a matter for conjecture at the time of this writing.

In the present question, however, there is no known sexually transmittable disease per se, there is merely a concern about high risk sexual behavior. In this scenario, information about sexual behavior is vested with confidentiality, and the therapist has no authority to breach confidentiality because of a perceived high risk of infection of another person. Given legal trends, however, the laws of the jurisdiction should be checked for this and related matters.

The logical approach would be to counsel each member of the couple, presumably individually at first and eventually the couple together, about all clinically significant aspects of keeping information from each other (e.g., as relevant to mutual respect and trust), promiscuous sexual behavior, and the risk of sexually transmittable diseases.

What needs to be stated in a form for authorizing the release of confidential or privileged communication?

The underlying legal principle is informed consent. The exact elements of informed consent are determined by the particular situation; for example, evidence that the client knew the purpose served and the possible positive and negative consequences resulting from the release of the information; authorized the particular receiver of the information (e.g., by name or facility); was aware of what was contained in the records or information that would be released; and had mental competency and was voluntarily granting the waiver of confidentiality (e.g., there was neither mental duress nor undue influence from the therapist). The release should provide for a time frame for the authorization and a means by which it can be rescinded (e.g., orally or in writing). Usually a release form need not be notarized or witnessed, but having these supportive sources is helpful for confirming that the release was executed in a proper manner.

I hate to be bothered by repeatedly asking a client to sign a release of confidential information form. A physician with whom I have professional contacts routinely has a patient sign several blank release forms; then whenever the patient calls and says send my records to so-and-so, the physician dates and fills in the form. Is this a reasonable solution?

Having blanket release forms is foolish, and does not conform to the legal underpinnings for informed consent. As revealed in the preceding question and answer, various elements of contemporary knowledge have to be accommodated at the time that the authorization is granted. Having previously signed release forms falls far short of the legal standards. "Being bothered" is no justification for neglecting strict adherence to the legal requirements for informed consent.

If I receive a subpoena for a client's records and he or she tells me that I should not send the records anyway, what should I do?

A therapist has no choice but to respond to a subpoena issued in his or her name. The type of response does, however, vary with the client's preferences.

For all of the following options, it is preferred that every contact be done in writing and sent by certified mail. This allows the therapist to document that he or she was attempting to honor the legal system as well as to safeguard the client, and that proper information was sent to and received by the particular source.

If the subpoena was issued by the client's attorney, it may not be mandatory to get the client's express approval to release the records. An attorney has a fiduciary duty to the client and, in a sense, steps into the client's shoes for this matter. Regardless, it is certainly prudent legally and wise clinically to contact the client to obtain written approval to release the records, even to the client's attorney.

Assuming that the subpoena is proper and the client does not want the therapist to release records or other confidential information, the therapist should inform the client or the client's attorney that unless timely authorization to honor the subpoena is given, the client should file a motion to quash the subpoena.

A motion to quash a subpoena, also known as a motion for a protective order, affords the client an opportunity to appear (usually represented by counsel) before the court to explain why the therapist's records should not have to be provided.

In the event that the client or his or her attorney does not move forthrightly on this request, the therapist cannot assume that the records must be released anyway. The therapist must still, however, respond to the subpoena.

There are two options. The first, and usually the most practical, is to contact the attorney who issued the subpoena and indicate that the therapist respects and wishes to cooperate fully with the judicial process, but is duty bound to uphold the client's right to claim privileged communications for the records; and, since the client will not approve release of the information (i.e., expressly waive objection to the therapist's honoring the subpoena), the therapist respectfully requests that the opposing attorney file a motion to compel the therapist (as opposed to a motion for contempt of court against the therapist). Here again, the parties, usually through their attorneys, have the opportunity to persuade the court as to why the therapist should or should not be compelled to produce the records or reveal other confidentiality. Needless to say, it is certainly better for the therapist to be responding to a court order relevant to a motion to compel, as opposed to having to face a personalized motion for contempt of court for failing to respond properly to the subpoena.

In the rare event that the attorney issuing the subpoena will not agree to a motion to compel, the therapist must, regrettably, step forward and submit a motion to quash the subpoena (or a motion for a protective order) on behalf of the client's possible right to confidentiality. Here the therapist (advisedly with an attorney) must inform the court that the therapist respects and wants to cooperate fully with the judicial process, but because of the client's refusal to authorize releasing the information or take other legal action, the therapist respectfully submits the matter to the court to decide.

In all of these options, whatever the court orders must be accepted and acted upon unreservedly. By common law and often by statute (e.g., the rules of evidence, civil procedure, and/or criminal procedure), a client who is a party to a legal action may have no assured confidentiality for information that would otherwise be privileged (e.g., psychotherapy records). Therefore, and along with the presumption that justice is usually best served by having all relevant and material information potentially available as evidence for the legal proceedings, the court will commonly be hesitant to maintain confidentiality (i.e., grant a motion for a protective order) for records relevant to a party to a legal action.

When dealing with this complex issue, the therapist should not, in any way, try to become a legal advocate of the interests of the client, except for the singular matter of whether or not the records or other information should or should not be released in response to the subpoena. In other words, the therapist should not become embroiled in the merits of the issues being dealt with in the legal proceedings. The therapist is involved only to provide professional information to the trier of fact (the judge or the jury), and is not there to play quasi-lawyer.

If I saw a husband and wife for therapy, both together and individually, they file for a divorce, and the attorney for one of them sends me a subpoena for the records, what do I have to send?

By common law, when a husband and wife have a conjoint therapy session, what was said by one is not protected by confidentiality from the other who was present. Nonetheless, some jurisdictions have laws to the contrary, such as requiring approval of all involved persons before records are released.

The problem is often that the therapist will also have individual sessions with one or both of the spouses. Any information revealed by one spouse out of the presence of the other, by whatever medium (e.g., verbal, written, face-to-face, telephone, etc.), is potentially confidential. Therefore, if information was obtained in a session involving the therapist and one spouse, the response to the subpoena of records is subject to the various issues and options set forth in the preceding question and answer. Whether contained in written records or presented in oral testimony, information derived from a single client must either be authorized by that client or be predicated upon a court order.

Obviously a treatment plan that involved both couple and individual sessions can carry the risk of the therapist revealing something, say during a deposition, that presumably was not confidential between clients, only to have one of the clients later allege that the revelation had, in fact, been based on an individual session and should not have been revealed without his or her express approval. Therefore, it is always prudent to get a comprehensive waiver of confidentiality or a court order that would embrace any and all information and regardless of what legal form (e.g., documents, deposition, or courtroom testimony).

Incidentally, the commonplace (but unwise) practice of keeping all marital and family therapy records in the same file can create a problem. For example, the notes for a conjoint session might appear on the same page as notes for an individual session. In this event and lacking the necessary authorization, it is quite appropriate to photocopy the record, use a razor blade to excise the protected section, and then make another photocopy of the altered page (NOTE: This is better than simply trying to use a felt-tip marker to mask words, since the lettering is prone to bleed through the masking ink later). If this is done, there should be no subterfuge or denial that certain material was removed from the copies (and, of course, the original unaltered copy is retained), with the explanation that this was solely to protect the client's right to confidentiality.

If an attorney subpoenas "any and all records" for a client, and the client endorses my releasing the records, do I have to send everything that I have in the file?

Generally speaking, a proper subpoena, especially with the client's authorization, means just what it says, "any and all records."

Some therapists object to providing test protocols or answer sheets, thinking that this would be a violation of copyright. Under the fair use doctrine of the Copyright Act, the routine copying of health care records, including forms that are copyrighted, does not constitute a violation of copyright. (I am somewhat bewildered by the number of therapists who try to avoid releasing test records for this reason, yet think nothing of making multiple copies of answer sheets or other test materials to avoid the expense of purchasing them from the publisher!)

Some therapists object to providing handwritten notes, often reasoning that "since I have my own form of shorthand, they have no meaning to anyone other than myself" or "these notes were made for my personal use, not for the use of the client or anyone else." Neither of these two reasons is acceptable. Keep in mind that but for the treatment of the client, no records would have been made in the first place; the purpose of records includes conveying meaning for the benefit of the client to other sources. Therefore, records must adequately communicate to benefit the client, and there is no such thing as a record prepared about a client that was intended only for the therapist's use.

An illegible or incomprehensible shorthand record had better be meaningful to an outside source or else the therapist quite likely has failed to meet the prevailing minimum standard for the profession relevant to keeping records. As for being illegible or fragmented, it would seemingly be appropriate to have the records typed or clarified, indicating that the supplement was made to contribute meaning to the legal process (and knowing that this is, potentially, an admission against interest for the therapist, namely that the records had been inadequate or faulty in their initial form). If this is done, a copy of the original records should accompany the supplemented version and the therapist can anticipate having to answer for this corrective strategy and justify that the amended version is, in fact, consonant with the substance of the original version.

If the preparation of the records for responding to the subpoena triggers recall of certain facts, ideas, or opinions that were not contained in the original documentary version, it is potentially proper for the therapist to prepare a supplemental or augmentation report. A newly prepared report must be dated in the present and acknowledge that the information therein resulted from the therapist's memory being refreshed. This augmentive strategy will likely lead to an inquiry during the legal process, such as an attorney asking the therapist during a deposition to justify deciding to provide additional information (i.e., was it proper clinical concern or improper legal advocacy by the therapist).

Between now and a deposition a couple of weeks ago, I have somehow lost some of the records for the case. Tomorrow I am scheduled for a follow-up deposition, and do not know how to explain the missing records. What do I say?

Just stand fast with the truthful answer; this is always the best policy. The records known to exist have inexplainably been misplaced. Knowing many offices, it seems likely that, for some reason, the missing sheets got out of the folder and were misfiled or put in the wastebasket by mistake. Whatever the reason, so be it.

As mentioned in the preceding question and answer, and in a later one about records destroyed by natural disaster, the therapist can use memory to reconstruct records or write a summary of them. Of course, this new document should be identified and dated accordingly.

The dilemma in this scenario underscores the importance of always maintaining a fail-safe system to preserve records. While perhaps lost by human error, such as by a file clerk, the therapist is still the focal point for possible legal liability.

Sometimes there are things in a client's records that I believe should not be involved in litigation. It might be damaging to the client. Can I just eliminate those records or pretend they do not exist?

As discussed in various other questions and answers, the therapist must never alter, destroy, or withhold records by personal preference (only by court order). Also, the therapist has no justification for either promoting or hampering litigation.

A therapist has societal endorsement for advocating mental health, not legal outcomes. Once a client is in litigation, the advocacy of mental health does not allow making judgments to influence the legal outcome.

For example, a client's mental health will likely be impacted negatively upon by imprisonment, but the therapist would not be allowed to exclude information that would lead to conviction and imprisonment under the guise that this was advocating the client's mental health interests. Absurd as this may be, it is dismaying how often a mental health therapist inappropriately and illegally deals with information under the self-aggrandizing delusion that it is justified by advocating mental health interests.

I was treating a young adult who committed suicide. My deceased client's parents want a copy of the treatment records and wish to meet with me and discuss the therapy that I had provided. How should I handle this request?

When a person dies, by whatever reason, his or her legal rights do not automatically extinguish. Therefore, no matter how well meaning the parents may be or the sympathy and wish to be supportive that is engendered in the therapist, there can be no release of confidential information without proper legal authorization.

While jurisdictions vary, it may be that the laws for the particular jurisdiction do, in fact, allow (or require) that a therapist release records or provide confidential information to a medical examiner for purposes of an autopsy. The law for the same jurisdiction may or may not extend the authorization to law enforcement personnel or for litigation purposes.

If there is any doubt, the therapist should consult with an attorney familiar with the laws applicable to the particular jurisdiction. Whatever the potentially unauthorized source, be it parents or law enforcement officers, there can presumably be a petition to the court to obtain authorization.

There is no definite ethical responsibility to meet with the parents of a deceased client. In fact, it is probably risky to hold such a meeting, because human nature often leads the grieving person(s) to seek solace through blaming others. Well-meaning parents seeking emotional support might eventually shift to alleging legally that the therapist was guilty of failing to take reasonable professional steps to prevent the suicide. As a rule of thumb, it is best to refer relatives of a deceased client to another therapist for grief therapy.

I have been in practice for a number of years, and have boxes of files all around my office suite and my home. The boxes are not well indexed, and by this time it is almost impossible to find an old file when I look for it. In fact, I seldom need to find an old file, and when I do, the information is so outdated that it is useless. When can I get rid of all these records? How do I have to keep records?

As mentioned previously, the laws for the jurisdiction in which the therapist practices may contain a mandatory time frame for retaining records. Also, certain professional associations deal with these matters in their codes of ethics; of course ethical guidelines do not supersede the applicable laws.

There are two important issues involved here. First, the standard of care requires maintaining records in a manner that makes them useful. To have allowed the records to become so disorganized that retrieval is difficult or impossible is potentially a violation of standards and actionable under law. Second, deciding when to get rid of records involves more than simply the minimum length of time specified by either law or ethics. The answer will depend on when the records are of no significance to either the clinical benefit of the client or risk management benefit of the therapist. Legal action sometimes occurs years after the last contact with the plaintiff. Thus, before discarding any records, the therapist should ponder the existing risk of a legal action for which the records would be needed for defensive purposes. The comment "the information is so outdated that it is useless" is more easily said than proven. It may end up that information from years ago has contemporary usefulness for legal purposes, whether for the benefit of the client or the therapist.

Believe it or not, a storm resulted in water damage to a number of client files that I had stored in a rented garage. The records are all caked together, and are now unusable. How do I handle this situation?

Unless a governmental regulatory agency has adopted a rule on this matter (which has, in fact, been done for the aftermath of certain natural disasters), the therapist can attempt to reconstruct any records that memory or other data sources will accommodate. If this is done, the dating of the reconstructed records should be noted. More likely, the therapist will be left to counter any future need or request for records with an affidavit about the loss of the records. The possibility of destruction of records by fire or "acts of God" justifies concern. Consideration should be given, for example, to purchasing file cabinets that maximize protection of the records.

Recall the previously used slogan, "An ounce of prevention is worth a pound of cure." One weekend, a national mental health association had a fire in its office suite that destroyed a massive amount of information. By regular practice, every Friday afternoon a prudent employee had made backup computer disks of a significant amount of the records and kept the disks at home, thereby saving valuable records.

Theft also merits concern. Given the nature of the cases served by the therapist, locked files and other security measures are essential. One office assistant was so worried about the documentary evidence contained in the file for a highly emotional case that she made a photocopy of everything in the file and kept it at her home. Under mysterious circumstances, the file in the office with the original documents disappeared, and was believed to be stolen. The defendant's glee changed abruptly when the photocopied file was produced, and the legal action went forward.

I am moving across the country, but will still be in practice. Should I send the records back to the clients whom I have seen here?

Whenever there is a change of location, the therapist is obligated to make a reasonable effort to be sure that past clients can obtain records in the future. The laws of certain jurisdictions prescribe how this must be done, such as by running notices in the newspaper.

Depending on the magnitude and nature of the clientele, direct contacts by letter (e.g., a mailed announcement of the new address) is one option. Of course clients move as well, and this approach may be ineffective, especially for clients served several years in the past.

It is also feasible to have another practitioner, such as a former associate, assume protection and control of the records and keep them locally. If reasonable precautions to maintain confidentiality are taken, the associate becomes an agent of the therapist and there should be no breach of confidentiality.

Given that one of the purposes for retaining records is risk management benefits for the benefit of the therapist, records should not be returned to the clients.

I plan to retire from practice. I expect that I will stay in the area, but do not want contacts with past clients. What should I do about the case records?

The preceding answer applies fully to this question as well. It is probably best to announce retirement, either by newspaper or direct mail, and to designate a keeper of the records (again, implementing reasonable safeguards for preservation of confidentiality). Again, some jurisdictions have laws (e.g., rules promulgated by licensing agencies) about this issue; better talk to an attorney.

While I fantasize that I will live forever, I know that someday I will die. At my death, what happens to records for my clients?

Human nature seems to preclude effective planning for death. This propensity has led some jurisdictions to pass laws, such as rules concomitant to professional licensing statutes, that prescribe how records must be handled after the death of the therapist. Commonly this involves notice of the disposition of the records by publication in a newspaper for the community in which the therapist practiced.

Regardless of any legal prescription per se, the therapist should make arrangements for someone, preferably another professional in the same mental health discipline or an attorney, to be caretaker of the records after the therapist's death. This arrangement should be in writing and could be included in testamentary documents (e.g., a will). Since there is the possibility, at least in some jurisdictions, that a legal action could be taken against the estate of the decedent-therapist, the records should not be destroyed. Further, the rights of the clients necessitate that the records must not fall into disarray or be opened to nonprofessional or unauthorized access.

I once looked at a house for possible purchase. It belonged to the widow of the town's physician. On commenting to her about the garage full of file cabinets, she said they were her deceased husband's records for patients and how, given her age and frail health, she hoped the purchaser of the house would take care of the records. Not a very professional outcome was it?

7

Business Issues

Almost every issue discussed so far has revealed changes in mental health services, as well as changes in the public policies and laws that relate to them. It is an understatement to assert that one of the greatest challenges to today's mental health practitioner is to adapt to the profound changes that have occurred and will continue to occur.

Being considered an integral member of the health care system is a change that most mental health practitioners have welcomed. As a result, the public has become more aware of the professional status and the important contribution of mental health practitioners. Stated simply, employment opportunities have expanded and incomes have increased.

When mental health professionals became part of the health care industry, however, they discovered that they had to conduct their practices according to business principles.

Being an astute business person is difficult enough, but interweaving the objectives and values of health care and business, which are sometimes contradictory, is exceptionally difficult. This blend calls for an unfailing altruistic commitment to the client, and an unabashed self-serving effort to succeed as a commercial operation. Without the latter, maintaining a successful practice is impossible.

When increased legal liability is added to the clinical–commercial mix, it is obvious that the mental health practitioner must possess well-honed business skills. Unfortunately, professional training programs have generally ignored or minimized preparation of trainees for the business aspects of practice. This chapter will highlight the sorts of business knowledge and skills that are necessary for a successful mental health practice, with special emphasis on how effective business operations will provide benefits to the client and legal safeguards for the practitioner.

Where can I get a book of forms for the business aspects of my mental health practice?

Some publishers market compilations of forms relevant to clinical practice. The prospect of finding a form that is ideal for a business aspect is minimal. Just as a treatment plan must be tailored to the particular client, every business document must be tailored to the issues and conditions unique to the particular mental health practice.

Often the notion of "finding a form" is rooted in having heard that attorneys use forms and wanting to avoid paying an attorney for legal services. It is true that attorneys have access to all sorts of forms, but the standards for legal practice hold that selecting a form (from among many possible forms) must rely on legal judgment. Even more importantly, editions of the selected form are available to meet the needs specific to the particular law client.

The conscientious attorney will accommodate the client's wish to minimize legal fees. That is, the attorney's use of a form should be reflected in the billing, with the fee being in accordance with the service actually provided.

Can you send me an employment contract that I can change around for each new associate?

No, an attorney should not send a therapist an employment contract to change around for each new associate. This would be like a therapist being asked to send copies of a psychological test to an employer with no training as a mental health professional to use as he or she wanted for testing employees. It is a matter of professional standards, and necessary to safeguard the consumer, that such contracts be individually tailored.

As reflected in the preceding question and answer about forms, any business or legal document must be individually tailored and involves legal expertise. By providing a form for adoption by a nonattorney, an attorney would be potentially accommodating an unnecessary risk for the parties to such an ill-thought out agreement.

A therapist looking for an employment contract that can be used with various mental health practitioners without legal advice is courting problems. Every employment arrangement should be unique to the employer and the employee, and it seems doubtful that there is, or could there be, a form that is universally applicable to the employment of therapists.

While keeping costs down is good business, it is equally good business to be willing to pay certain costs that will enhance the quality of operations. Well-drafted legal documents are essential to good business. In this competitive and litigious era, supportive professional services, such as from an attorney or accountant, are essential.

Can I avoid social security, worker's compensation, and unemployment compensation taxes by calling my associates "Independent Contractors?"

The title attached to an associate in the workplace has little or no relevance to whether or not a worker is an employee or an independent contractor. What is legally required is satisfying the criteria set forth by the Internal Revenue Service (as well as, perhaps, a state revenue office). The criteria are available in Internal Revenue Regulation 31.3401.

As has been well publicized in this health care reform era, there is great governmental concern for employers' paying employee benefits, even for part-time employees. No one is above the law, and failure to pay employee benefits can certainly not be explained away by devious means, such as trying to use a title other than "employee."

It seems probable that the propriety of independent contractor status will be markedly decreased in the near future.

A long-time friend and I are thinking about going into practice together. We sense that we should have some sort of partnership agreement. How should we go about it?

Any business should operate by well-defined legal documents. Considering a practice with a long-time friend creates no exemption from the risks attendant to being in business with another (lesser known) person. It might even be that friendship leads to the parties' overlooking certain conditions that merit legal consideration; that is, the emotional dimension of friendship might lead to ignoring the obvious, which would be detected readily by objective legal scrutiny.

The term *partnership* may or may not be the form of business entity that is most appropriate for a practice. In point of fact, a partnership carries certain liabilities that are not present in a corporation. For example, all things being commonplace, if there is a debt and/or legal judgment against a partnership, and one partner has little or no money, the other partner(s) might be required to pay a disproportionately large portion of the debt and/or judgment from personal assets. Whereas in a corporation, again all things being commonplace, debts and/or judgments (excluding malpractice judgments) can seldom be levied against personal assets; the lien or collection will be confined to the corporate assets. Therefore, the selection of a business entity must be based on legal information for the circumstances unique to the practice.

Once a business entity has been selected, the legal documents will follow, with idiosyncratic considerations and provisions. Whatever may be contained in the legal documents (e.g., the rights and duties of the officers, directors, and shareholders), there should be planning for the dissolution. That may sound bizarre, but much like a prenuptial agreement between two persons who are coming into a marriage with assets earned previously, therapists should go into a business relationship with a contractual understanding about how their association will be terminated, whenever that may occur. Many lawsuits between therapists over business issues come at the point of breakup and could have been avoided, to everyone's benefit, by a prescribed legal solution from the onset.

I think it looks pretty spiffy when I see PA after a practitioner's name. How do I know when I should become a professional corporation?

"Pretty spiffy" might be good for one's ego, but it is a bad reason to form a professional service corporation (PC) or association (PA). Creating any sort of a business entity should be determined by a thorough analysis of operations and finances, and predicated on business planning and information from an accountant and an attorney.

There is no one formula for deriving either the need for or type of a particular business entity. Regardless of how clear-cut that information, there is always a managerial prerogative that can only be exercised by the therapist, i.e., the business principal.

Commonly, adopting a business entity, such as a corporation, is justified by using the legally established entity as a way of defining the rights and obligations of the investors and the manner in which the business operations will be conducted. Also, the amount of revenues may point toward adopting a particular entity because of tax or investment opportunities that would not be available otherwise.

The professional service corporation or PA is, generally speaking, used to accommodate interests aligned with professionalism. For example, the PA, as a business entity is usually available only to persons who hold a license from the state in which the business will be conducted. State laws vary; some states say only practitioners licensed in the same discipline can be shareholders in a professional service corporation, whereas some other states allow a mixture of licensed disciplines to be eligible for shareholder status.

Since each state has its unique laws, both by statute and case determinations, this entire matter requires thorough legal counsel based on the laws governing the jurisdiction in which the therapist practices.

I have been told that if I incorporate as a PA, I cannot be sued in malpractice. Should I incorporate?

The question is apparently referring to the so-called "corporate shield." Usually being a properly registered corporation allows liability to extend only to corporate assets. Thus, if the corporation incurred large debts, say for computer and telecommunications systems, and the purchases were made "for the corporation" (i.e., no personal surety) and the corporation had to dissolve, the legal judgments and liens obtained by the creditors could only be placed on the assets of the corporation.

Some states have laws that allow a professional service corporation to fashion a perimeter of liability that has relevance to clinical services. For example, the law may say that a practitioner operating as a professional service corporation has malpractice liability for only his or her personal conduct and/or the conduct of those for whom there is a supervisory duty. Thus, if there were, say, multiple practitioners housed in the same facility, there would be a potential limit to the vicarious liability imposed on a practitioner for allegedly wrongful conduct or malpractice by others.

Nonetheless, there is never an impenetrable corporate shield from liability for professional malpractice. For example, if two practitioners, each with PA status, are both involved in the service chain for a given client, an allegation of negligent conduct might be directed at both of them, notwithstanding the professional service corporation issue.

As with so many of the questions about business, a particular jurisdiction can have unique twists, and legal counsel relevant to the jurisdiction in which the therapist practices is essential.

My landlord wants me to sign a lease "personally," as opposed to in the name of our clinic. What are the implications?

The corporate shield has a place in the operations of a therapy practice. For example, assume that a therapist had a professional service corporation and entered into a long-term lease for an office suite; and the commitment was "for the Corporation." If the rent (and other overhead expenses) proved to be beyond payment possibility and the professional service corporation were dissolved without substantial assets, it is likely that there would be no way for the landlord to collect unpaid rents for the remainder of the lease. Of course many creditors, like a landlord, are savvy to the protections afforded by the corporate shield, and will require that a lease or debt have other surety, such as the incorporated therapist's signing both "for the Corporation and Personally," thereby making it possible for the creditor to reach to the therapist's personal (noncorporate) assets in the event of nonpayment.

NOTE: There are other legal considerations when there is an abrogation of a valid lease, as well as nonpayment of other debts. Therefore, the foregoing comments are to clarify the corporate shield principle, and should not be considered a thorough explanation of the debt–liability issues. Again, the laws of the jurisdiction would prevail.

If I incorporate, I gather I will get a number of tax benefits, and that I can make all sorts of deductions from my income, including deducting my daughter's college expenses by paying them out of corporate funds. This sounds too good to be true. Can I deduct her college expenses?

First, being incorporated does allow certain tax options. Establishing the professional service corporation or PA to accommodate professional interests is buttressed by the so-called "Subchapter S" election for reporting to the Internal Revenue Services. In brief, the Subchapter S election means that instead of corporate taxes, with all their different rules, the taxpayer can elect to continue to file according to individual taxpayer rules, yet still be a corporation. For the therapy practice, short of high earnings and operational complexity, the Subchapter S election is usually preferred, subject to accounting or legal analysis to the contrary.

As for paying a daughter's college expenses, the therapist asking the question is correct: it is too good to be true. However, if the daughter were an employee of the corporation and the corporation made educational benefits available to all employees, a deduction might be proper.

Another practitioner and I have had a corporation for several years. We no longer get along well, and believe that we should probably split up. How do we go about it?

To paraphrase a religious statement, "As the state giveth, so can the state taketh away." Just as the state creates a corporation by registration, it can dissolve a corporation. If the owners of the corporation agree on the dissolution, they can implement a voluntary dissolution. State laws vary, but commonly the corporation must petition for a dissolution. Some states, however, automatically dissolve a corporation if a periodic renewal fee is not paid in a timely manner.

If the owners of the corporation disagree about the dissolution, say because they cannot agree on how existing accounts receivable or debts will be divided, it is usually possible to petition for an involuntary dissolution. A conservator may be appointed by the court. Assets and liabilities have to be reported and resolutions fashioned.

There have been bitter legal battles between mental health practitioners, of which some were surprisingly soon after what seemed to be a "perfect marriage" of professional interests. There is a popular song, performed by the Carpenters, that warns, "breaking up is hard to do." Indeed, it is. This is another reason why no professional business should be formed without wise analysis, planning, and documentation. The latter could, of course, include provisions for dissolving the corporation. These provisions should be formulated at the onset when there is a more sane state of affairs than would be the case during the "divorce" process.

I want to start practicing alone here in the same town. My partner says that he will buy my share of our corporation, but for just a nominal fee, basically the value of the office furniture and equipment. Is this fair?

There is no surefire way of deriving what is or is not a "fair" buy out figure. Accountants have a plethora of formulas that can be applied to evaluating a business for sale, which may offer ideas or guidelines that are potentially applicable to a mental health practice. Regardless, a considerable degree of subjectivity will remain.

The "good will" or "blue sky" value that so often constitutes a significant portion of the value of a business is seldom distinct for a mental health practice. The nature of therapy tends to align good will with a particular therapist and contradicts a blue sky value for the business name per se. There are, however, exceptions.

For example, if the mental health practice was known as the "Psychological Associates of Omigosh" or some other undistinguished (generic) name, as opposed to a distinctive name for a clinic, there would likely be minimal good will or blue sky value. Or if the professionals owning the practice had their personal names in its trade name, the blue sky value would be lessened. If the name of the practice is going to be abandoned, all name value would be eliminated.

If the practice, however, has contracts to provide service, say to an employee assistance program or other third-party payment source, and income therefrom was virtually assured, there is a value to which each owner has a rightful share. This means that payment for simply the "office furniture and equipment" would likely be unfair—that is, the therapist selling his or her ownership rights deserves a share of the value of the contracts, proportionate to his or her investments.

As emotions rise during the divorce of business partners, notions about values of the business too often become unrealistic. As a rule of thumb, the would-be seller should ask: "If I were buying the same sort of business interests, what would I be willing to pay." Much to the disappointment of the therapist who has, in fact, made a tremendous investment of time, energy, and finances into developing the practice, the answer is most often: "I would not pay much."

Why this negative answer? Because the would-be buyer who can afford to purchase a practice usually has developed a set of professional skills, and quickly realizes that the selling practitioner's departure from the marketplace will make it possible for the newcomer to pursue the clientele that were formerly attracted to the practice. The would-be buyer calculates what would be necessary to capture the market, and often recognizes that within a fairly short period of time, say a few months (especially with the seller out of the competition), there is precious little that could actually be obtained from the seller that could not be obtained by hard work on one's own.

The calculations can become more refined. As one example, assume a seasoned practitioner operates the XYZ Clinic and employs three lesser trained associates. By analysis, it is apparent that clients are attracted to the XYZ Clinic because of the professional reputation of the senior person, and the associates do not have an employment contract with a noncompetition clause. Thus, if the practice were sold, the buyer might find that referrals would diminish considerably because of the personal absence of the departed senior therapist and the associates would exit to another practice, perhaps even soliciting the clients served at the XYZ Clinic to follow them elsewhere. So what is left to be sold? Only the office furniture and equipment remain for a buyer.

I am leaving our group practice and have been planning to take my clients with me. My partners say that the clients belong to the practice. I say I have an ethical responsibility to keep treating my clients. Who is right?

It all depends on the legal structure of the practice. A fiduciary duty may preclude a departing partner's taking clients seen in the group practice.

Assuming that all partners were co-owners of the practice, and even if there were varying amounts of ownership between partners (i.e., one partner owned a larger portion of the practice than the others), each partner should have a fiduciary duty to practice. Certain business entities, such as a corporation, would find special legal enforcement for the fiduciary duty issue.

By fiduciary duty, each partner (or corporate director) is legally bound to promote the business interests of the other partners (or corporate directors) and the organization. There can be no undue self-serving action at the expense of the others. The fiduciary duty also commonly extends to employees, albeit the extent of duty has been a frequent subject of litigation between employers and employees.

Further, a prudent, well-planned practice will operate with prescriptive and proscriptive legal documents, such as a shareholders' agreement, by-laws, employment contracts, and so on. These legal documents, with the force of business and contract laws, can determine whether or not the clientele is protected.

While state laws can vary on the subject, it is common to consider information about clientele to be "trade secrets" potentially protected by unfair competition laws. Also, noncompetition agreements can negate pirating clientele from a former employer.

Some mental health practitioners try to assert that professional ethics allow them to take their clients along, regardless of business interests. It should always be remembered that ethical practices are not laws, and laws are always superior to ethical practices, no matter how well-intentioned the latter may be. While it is true that a client cannot be sold like a chattel and the client always has the right to seek professional services from whomever he or she wishes to see, it is a legal fact that a practitioner can be reasonably restrained from unfair competition, which could include, for example, solicitation of clients from the practice in which the departing therapist was a partner, co-owner, or employee.

The repeated caveat about needing business planning and legal agreements prior to initiating a practice is applicable again. The issue of what happens to clients when a therapist departs should definitely be established by contractual agreement from the onset of affiliation or employment, and must be consonant with the laws of the jurisdiction.

I have been a postdoctoral trainee for the last two years, in order to quality for licensure in my state. I passed the examination, and now intend to strike out on my own. My supervisor-employer tells me that our initial agreement keeps me from practicing in the

same town or continuing to see or contact the clients whom I saw during my internship. Is this legal?

While each state has unique laws for noncompetition, it is common to legally uphold noncompetition agreements that are reasonable. As noted in the preceding question and answer, unfair competition laws protect certain trade secrets, which can include information about clientele. Noncompetition laws usually require a reasonable definition according to clientele, type of services provided, geographical considerations, and duration of the noncompetition.

For example, if a noncompetition agreement said that a departed employee could not practice his or her profession anywhere in the state, and the employer only drew clients from, say, one county, it is unlikely that the agreement would be upheld by a court. Likewise, if the noncompetition agreement were for a long period of time, it would be less likely to be upheld than if it were for a short period of time. All of the variables in a noncompetition agreement are subject to the statutory and case law of the jurisdiction governing the agreement.

As reflected with previous questions and answers, the noncompetition issue should be addressed in writing and in accord with the governing laws from the onset of employment or training. Given the pronounced consequences of having or failing to have a noncompetition agreement, it is amazing how many employers neglect the issue and how many employees and trainees enter into a noncompetition agreement without realizing to what they are agreeing.

During my most recent employment, I worked for a percentage of the fees collected for my services by the senior practitioner. We have parted company and are on reasonably good terms. However, my ex-boss does not want to pursue collections from some of the overdue accounts. I believe that I should be allowed to take over the accounts. How should we handle this problem?

It depends on the employment arrangement. The prudent and wise business person, whether the employer or employee, will settle this issue before beginning the employment relationship.

If there is no written agreement with relevant terms, the matter is rife for litigation. For example, if there is no contractual arrangement, the departed employee could assert that payment was due whenever fees are collected for the services that he or she provided, regardless of the passage of time (e.g., years later). On the other hand, the employer could assert that no departed employee could reasonably expect to receive compensation whenever the payments trickled in—and besides, the extended period required the employer to incur collection expenses that were not part of the understanding during the course of employment and these additional collection expenses should be deducted from any funds to which the ex-employee lays claim.

Human nature being what it is, selective memory may operate (especially in an emotionalized conflict situation), and there may be differing views about what was embraced by the verbal agreement. Obviously the only solution is a proper contractual agreement from the onset of the employment relationship.

Another therapist, with a practice much stronger than mine, has offered to send cases to me, but wants a percentage of what I collect from these clients. I believe that this is illegal fee splitting. Is there a way to make this kind of arrangement legitimate?

There are many possible nuances to this scenario, and more details would be necessary to answer definitely. Most basically, there is such a thing as "unlawful fee splitting." The Federal Trade Commission has, however, declared that certain shared business ventures between professionals, including therapists, should not be precluded by codes of ethics.

State statutes likely define the matter. For example, some licensing laws will call for disciplinary action against those licensed mental health professions that have certain exchange of fees and referrals between practitioners. Florida Statute 491.009(2)(j) states that there will be potential disciplinary action against a licensee for:

> [P]aying a kickback, rebate, bonus, or other remuneration for receiving a patient or client, or receiving a kickback, rebate, bonus,

or other remuneration for referring a patient or client to another provider of mental health care services or to a provider of health care services or goods; referring a patient or client to oneself for services on a fee-paid basis when those services are already being paid for by some other public or private entity; or entering into a reciprocal referral agreement.

Further, if the funding for the mental health services comes from federal sources, there may be federal laws and/or concomitant rules that have to be considered.

As a rule of thumb, any payment–referral plan should: (1) be well defined; (2) be put in writing; (3) be in accord with state and federal laws and rules; (4) require that all persons receiving funds have a continued involvement with the case management; and (5) be reasonably known to all interested parties (such as the client and any third-party payment source).

It should be remembered that shared professional involvement will potentially mean that legal allegations against the treating therapist for malpractice may create vicarious liability for the referring therapist, notwithstanding the fact that he or she did not do the treatment per se. That is, since the referring therapist has a continued involvement (as well as monetary interest) in the treatment of the client, it could readily be asserted that he or she has a legal duty to reasonably safeguard and assure quality care for the client (especially if supervision was being provided to the treating therapist) and negligence by the treating therapist could potentially be imputed to the referring therapist. This matter is set forth as a warning that referral plans should be cautiously accepted. While generally there is no liability for simply referring a client to an independent practitioner, the liability arises for a shared enterprise.

I am always uneasy about discussing fees with a client, especially in the first few sessions. How do I overcome this reluctance?

There is no reason to be uneasy about talking about fees with a client, and numerous reasons why it should preface any professional services. Professional ethics have generally adopted the view that failing to discuss the financial aspects of treatment, preferably at the onset of service, could violate the ethical standards for the discipline.

Therapeutically, it is easy to recognize that a client who finds him- or herself in a treatment situation that involves a mounting financial obligation that cannot be met will surely experience negative effects. That is, the unpaid debt will, consciously or unconsciously, impact adversely on the client's psychological comfort and growth, as well as the therapist's motivation and helping qualities.

Overcoming reluctance to talk about financial issues should be easy, especially in this health care reform era when mental health services are unquestionably viewed as a business and part of the health care industry. Basically, the therapist should recognize that the professional service relationship is predicated on a so-called "economic exchange" principle, which holds that the client's coming for service justifies a quid pro quo for the therapist, namely in the form of the client's compliance with the treatment plan and payments according to an agreed upon financial arrangement.

Since having a clear pretreatment financial arrangement has evolved to being a matter of ethics, it is incontrovertible that failing to discuss the financial aspects of treatment in a timely manner is unprofessional and a potential breach of ethics. Therefore, the therapist must accept that it is a professional mandate and act accordingly.

I seem to have a significant number of clients who have trouble paying their bills. I have talked to other therapists, and I seem to have greater difficulty in getting paid than they do. Am I doing something wrong?

The word *wrong* can take on several connotations. As discussed earlier, it is commonplace and ethical to make the financial terms clear from the onset of service. Theoretically, it is generally believed that treatment efficacy is compromised by allowing the client to receive services that impose an undue financial burden. The client is prone to suffer a negative affective or defensive response, whether it is inappropriate guilt or sense of obligation or subservience; and the therapist is prone to have a negative reaction, such as sensing that he or she is being put upon unfairly by the client. In any event, the quality of treatment is lessened. Finally, the therapist cannot continue in practice without adequate financial compensation.

Before initiating ongoing treatment or services, there should be a definite financial arrangement, preferably in written contractual form. In this agreement, the mutual responsibilities should be stated, that is, what the therapist shall provide (e.g., a reasonable standard of care) and what the client's quid pro quo shall be (e.g., a certain payment for each session, acceptance of responsibility for payment regardless of whether or not third-party insurance payments are received, interest to be paid on overdue accounts, and adherence to the treatment plan).

Since the professional service relationship is predicated on exchange theory, meaning each party (the therapist and the client) provides the other with a benefit, it is illogical to attempt to provide services without a mutually satisfactory set of conditions for the relationship. As noted, professional associations recognize this principle, and have embraced it in codes of ethics. Regardless of humanitarian or "Ivory Tower" notions, public policy and laws for this health care reform era leave no doubt that mental health services are, in fact, part of the health care industry, and must be conducted accordingly. Therefore, sound business practices are mandatory, which will benefit both the client and the therapist.

Having a significant number of clients who fail to pay their accounts seemingly reflects an inadequate service delivery system. It is essential to carefully screen potential clients to assure that anyone accepted for professional services can fulfill the elements of the exchange theory model that is applied to professional services. To do otherwise is to be potentially unethical and unprofessional, and courting elevated legal liability and financial risks.

Can I charge a client for telephone conferences?

If the client agrees to the conditions for payment (and they are not void by public policy or illegal), the therapist can charge for any professional service. Whether for a telephone conference or any other professional service, the client should know ahead of time what will incur a charge, as well as payment arrangements (e.g., interest on overdue accounts).

As a rule of thumb, it seems logical and appropriate to impose a fee when the following three questions are answered in the affirmative. First, was the service for the principal benefit of the client? Second, did the service rely on the therapist's professional training and skills? Third, was the therapist potentially liable for what occurred (e.g., said or done) in the service? If the answer to each of these questions is "yes," a professional fee is justified. Certainly a substantive telephone conference could fulfill each of these criteria, thereby justifying a charge.

A telephone conference can be as important to treatment as any other service, and certainly merits a fee. A telephone conference should be handled like any other therapeutic services, with thoughtful responses, written notes for the clinical record, and a fee. For the therapist's personal welfare, certain structural issues should be honored, such as perhaps having the telephone conference scheduled ahead of time or establishing beforehand that the client will not expect the therapist to stop whatever else might be occurring, such as on a weekend, to enter into a telephone conference on the spur of the moment.

A special billing problem may arise when, for the welfare of the client, the therapist has to have a telephone conference with another health care provider (e.g., the client's family physician, a child-client's teacher, the client's attorney in a legal case). Since the client may not be able to give explicit approval for an unexpected or extratherapeutic telephone conference (but assuming proper authorization to release confidential information has been given), the policy for charging for these telephone conferences with other sources for the benefit of the client should be set forth in a policy statement, preferably as part of a written service agreement entered into by the client and the therapist at the beginning of the therapeutic relationship.

The billing problem comes not from the appropriateness of charging for a telephone conference, but from the fact that a third-party payment source (e.g., a health insurance carrier) might not cover this service and the client would have to make the payment in full. This potential nonreimbursement should be reckoned with at the onset of the treatment relationship, just like any other financial issue.

As might be assumed, there are certain telephone conferences for which a charge would not be appropriate; for example, simply talking to a client about a schedule change. If there is therapeutic substance, however, the fee would be appropriate. None of the foregoing should be interpreted as advocacy for substituting telephonic therapy for face-to-face therapy, albeit that electronic media are progressing in a manner that will justify continual reassessment of this issue.

I find expert testimony highly demanding, and not at all enjoyable. Can I charge a fee higher than my regular fee for therapy?

As with any professional service, a therapist is entitled to charge whatever is appropriate to his or her skills and the particular marketplace.

The term *price gouging* arises when a service recipient has no choice but to accept services from a particular source and the price is, therefore, elevated. This risk, along with not wanting to create an appearance of impropriety (see next paragraph), supports that it is unwise to raise the fee simply because there is dislike for being involved in legal proceedings.

Some jurisdictions have a set fee for expert testimony, which is often quite low. For example, one state statute allows the court to order a mere $10 per hour for expert testimony. If a judge learns that the therapist has raised his or her professional fee because of being displeased over having been called into the judicial system, there is the risk of the judge's considering the therapist's attitude or conduct to constitute an appearance of impropriety, and may enter an order with negative financial consequences for the therapist. In general, it is definitely best to have an established fee that remains the same for all professional services (at least as concerns forensic versus nonforensic contexts).

On several occasions, I have had to appear in court for a client. The attorney calling me to testify will tell me to clear, say one hour, and I have to allow travel time before and after the hour. All too often, when I get there, I end up sitting around in the courtroom for, say, a couple of hours, and then may testify for only twenty or thirty minutes. If I charge only for the time that I am actually testifying, I cannot afford to continue in practice. What is the fair way to charge a client for my time?

A therapist is allowed to charge for any time or service provided for the benefit of the client, as long as the charge is agreed upon (explicitly or implicitly) ahead of time by the client. A forensic contract, entered into by the client and therapist, at the onset of treatment should deal with the computation of and payment for time committed to legal matters.

One of the common responses from therapists is: "I had no idea the couple would divorce when I started treatment, so I saw no reason to talk about getting paid for my time in a court case." In this litigious era, it should be assumed that every client is a potential litigant, and the therapist could be brought into a legal fray regardless of his or her expectations or preferences.

All treatment should be prefaced by a payment arrangement, which clarifies charges if or when the therapist is drawn into a legal case because of the professional relationship with the client. The definitions should include time required for travel, waiting-in-the-courtroom time, telephone conferences and depositions with attorneys (regardless of which party's attorney calls or subpoenas the therapist), review of notes in preparation for testimony, and so on.

I have been subpoenaed to appear in court, and do not want to be involved in the case. How can I avoid it?

If a proper subpoena is issued (meaning, among other things, that the therapist is subject to the jurisdiction from which the subpoena emanates), and there has been no order to quash the subpoena, the therapist cannot avoid it—nor should the therapist try to avoid the authority of a proper subpoena. Every citizen must honor the laws, and the laws provide for subpoena power.

If a subpoena is received that the therapist believes is improper, a motion to quash can be filed. That is, the therapist can petition the court to deny legal authority to the subpoena. Stated differently, the court can order protection of the therapist.

If a client has privileged communication and the therapist is subpoenaed to produce the client's records or give a deposition or courtroom testimony about professional services to the client, the therapist should contact the client (perhaps through his or her attorney) and get express written approval to honor the subpoena. If the client does not approve, the client should be instructed to file a motion for a protective order, thereby allowing the court to decide whether the client's privileged communication should be upheld or denied. There are some circumstances that might necessitate the therapist's initiating the motion for a protective order on behalf of the client, which would assure that the therapist could not be faulted later by the client for alleged violation of privileged communication.

One of my clients was injured in an automobile accident and is suing the other driver, actually the automobile insurance company, and has incurred a large debt for my assessment and therapy services about which I will testify in the personal injury suit. My client does not have adequate funds to cover this debt. The client's attorney has offered me a so-called "letter of protection." Is this adequate for me to demand payment later on? What if the client loses the case?

A "letter of protection" is, more often than not, of minimal or no actual benefit. Even though the attorney for the client writes the letter, the attorney will not generally be liable personally for the debt. The debt is supposed to remain with the client.

With varying degrees of scruples, some attorneys will offer to write a letter of protection, wherein there is a precatory promise that the bill from the expert witness will be given "priority" or "consideration" in the event that the client gains a judgment. Of course there are some legal cases in which gaining a judgment does not produce any funds, e.g., having a judgment that the debtor can escape by having no attachable funds or discharge in bankruptcy.

Since the letter of protection from the attorney is seldom enforceable by contract law, the therapist may have to take legal action to get paid by the client (assuming that the client is financially able to cover the debt).

As for the "degrees of scruples" mentioned earlier, some attorneys have been known to contact the expert witness and say, in effect, "When I wrote you the letter of protection, the client was anticipating receiving $100,000, but since only $50,000 has been received, we are reducing all fees to experts by 50%—which you can either accept or get nothing voluntarily from my client." Obviously this is a crude (and unscrupulous?) attempt to coerce the expert witness into accepting a substantial reduction in a legitimately deserved fee.

With this scenario, many therapists tend to prefer to avoid a legal battle or to not alienate a client, and they recall the old adage, "A bird in the hand is worth two in the bush." They reason that if they do not settle for the reduced amount before it is dispersed, there may be no other funds available from which to gain a collection, and there would be the emotional and financial expense of litigation, bad public relations, and the risk of a retaliatory complaint to a regulatory agency or an ethics committee.

Then there is always the possibility that the client will not prevail in the litigation, and that no judgment will be gained. In this instance, all of the previously mentioned negative considerations are present, plus there is no money from which to gain even a reduced fee. In other words, the letter of protection ended up offering no protection.

Incidentally, for both ethical and legal reasons, a therapist should not work for a contingency fee, that is, a percentage of the recovery, if any. The therapist should work only for an established reasonable fee.

I have had several cases that unexpectedly ended up in court. For example, one of my psychotherapy clients was injured in a car accident, and could not keep working or afford treatment. The client's attorney contacted me, wanting me to keep seeing the client and give expert testimony in the personal injury suit. The attorney sent me a document titled "Letter of Protection," which

said "if a judgment is obtained, your bill for services will be considered for payment." This seems rather indefinite to me, but the attorney keeps trying to persuade me that I can trust the Letter of Protection. What should I do?

This matter has been dealt with in the preceding question and answer. Suffice it to say, a therapist does not have a legal duty to continue treating a client who cannot afford treatment. There is, of course, a duty to make a proper termination and referral. A new set of objectives, such as those created by a car accident, certainly goes beyond the meeting of the minds that took place when treatment was initiated. Further, being an expert witness is beyond the agreed upon role of being a therapist. Indeed, a modern trend for professional ethics and laws seems to be raising questions about the professional propriety of holding more than one role, such as being both a therapist and an evaluator, in a custody dispute.

While the therapist might be subpoenaed to appear and give fact testimony, there is no duty per se to provide expert testimony. Of course, if this matter were presented to the court and a judge ordered the therapist to testify as an expert, the order should be honored, along with a court-ordered arrangement for payment.

As for the "Letter of Protection," especially if it contains qualifying or conditional words, it offers little or no enforceable contractual duty for the client to make payments. The wise, prudent, and professionally correct position would be to not provide services of any kind that the client cannot afford or that the therapist is not otherwise motivated to provide, e.g., by benevolence.

When I have a client with health insurance who cannot afford to pay the unreimbursed portion of the bill, I tell them I will take just what the insurance pays. If a client's health insurance company pays, say 80%, and the client cannot afford to pay the unreimbursed portion of the bill, how about raising my fee so that the 80% would end up reimbursing me for my full fee? For example, if I regularly charge $100, the 80% reimbursement would mean that raising my fee to $125 would result in my getting my regular $100 fee.

In this health care reform age of concern about health care costs, the therapist should ponder how an auditor for an insurance company or a prosecuting attorney would react to this sort of arrangement. Stated bluntly, this idea is vulnerable to an allegation of wrongdoing, such as health care fraud. Telling the health insurance company that an elevated fee was charged to assure that the company's money covered the usual and customary (lower) fee because the client cannot afford to make the copayment would avoid fraud, but payment would be improbable.

There are some health insurance companies that will allow the practitioner to accept just what they pay, that is, no copayment is required of the client. Even then, elevating the fee above what is usual and customary is risky, and potentially comes under the heading of illegal gouging or fraud.

The solution is to be realistic about the business conditions in which today's therapist must operate, and to not resort to schemes that are potentially unethical or illegal. There should be complete disclosure of every bit of information that is relevant and material to the reimbursement issue.

Keep in mind that the therapist is not a party to the health insurance contract, it is between the insurance company and the insured client. If the client wants or needs better coverage (e.g., reimbursement at a higher rate), he or she can purchase that sort of policy. If the client cannot afford a better policy, there is no sound reason for the therapist to sense a duty to attempt to manipulate the situation or accept clients who are unable to meet the financial conditions to which the therapist is entitled.

Some pro bono or complimentary services may be appropriate for humanitarian reasons, but there is a limit to how much no-fee service can be provided by a therapist. Instead of becoming a benevolent agency, the therapist is better advised to engage in professional advocacy for improved financing of public mental health services.

I am licensed and typically eligible for reimbursement under health insurance policies. My associate, however, does not have a doctorate and is seldom, if ever, eligible for reimbursement. If my associate has a client with health insurance, I fill out the forms,

indicating that I did the therapy. Sometimes my associate does talk to me about the treatment or a particular client, but we do not have regular supervision, certainly not of every client who is treated by my associate. I know that certain other therapists in town do the same thing. However, my local attorney advised against this approach, but it seems all right to me. What am I missing?

This scenario returns to potential health care fraud. Full disclosure is axiomatic for all health care insurance issues.

An insurance form should accurately reveal (among other things) when, to whom, and what type of treatment was provided, and who actually provided the service. If an associate provided the service, it should be indicated. If the associate's services were supervised, say by the licensed professional, the supervisor should be indicated as well. Of course, there is a legal duty to actually provide the supervision, up to the reasonable and prevailing standards of the profession (or as specified by the health insurance contract or applicable laws). Keep in mind that, as the *respondeat superior*, the supervisor will likely be legally liable for every act committed or omitted by the associate, and supervision is, therefore, an essential safeguard for the supervisor.

There may well be other professionals in the community who do not exercise full disclosure, but "two wrongs don't make a right." If accused of health care fraud, there would be no assured defense from saying, "don't blame me, others do it too!"

I have encountered a drop in my referrals, and gather it is because more and more people have health insurance that requires them to see only practitioners designated by their carrier. I have been asked to affiliate with various Health Maintenance Organizations (HMOs) and Employee Assistance Programs (EAPs), but they seem to pay so poorly, I would rather not sign on with any of them. What are the legal concerns?

Managed health care systems commonly prescribe conditions to which an approved provider must adhere. The best treatment interests of certain clients may necessitate treatment qualities that are not accommodated by the restrictions imposed by the managed health care systems. Consequently, there is, indeed, a potential risk of allegations of malpractice or professional negligence imposed on the practitioner. Further, the agreements presented to therapists by the managed health care systems commonly require that the approved provider contractually agree to "hold harmless" and/or "indemnify" the managed health care system for any legal expenses resulting from allegations against the approved provider by a client.

What the managed health care systems are banking on (pun intended) is that the health care reform marketplace will require therapists to become approved providers. Thus, they aggressively pursue contracts, such as with employers, that will require service recipients, such as employees with a particular employer, to obtain services from an approved provider or pay for it out of their own pockets. The entire managed health care system is predicated on cost containment, otherwise known as low cost health care services.

Whether or not a therapist should accept clients from managed health care systems boils down to the strength of the practice. It is probable that clients referred by the managed health care systems will yield lower fees than, say, self-referred pay-as-you-go clients. However, the latter type of clients, those who will seek services independent of third-party payment plans, will likely be more difficult to attract than clients covered by restrictive policies, especially in this age of health care reform.

There is no simple solution. If the therapist decides that affiliation with managed health care systems is inevitable or unavoidable, an effort should be made to try to bring about leeway for tailoring the quality of service according to the needs of the particular client and to continue to cultivate other sources of income.

Once I start treating a client, is it unethical to terminate treatment because the client will not make payments?

It is not unethical per se to terminate treatment of a client who will not make payment. Remember that the professional service relationship is predicated on exchange theory, with mutual agreed upon benefits to the client and the therapist.

If the client abrogates his or her contractual duty to the therapist, there is certainly a legitimate basis for terminating treatment. The termination should, however, be accomplished in a tactful manner, with reasonable consideration to accommodating the client's mental health needs. Most commonly this means tapering off services (i.e., no abrupt termination), and implementing a referral for services elsewhere.

If the client rejects the idea of referral, the therapist can set forth a rationale that, since the client is no longer meeting the agreed upon conditions for the professional service relationship, there are factors that adversely impact on the quality of treatment and continuation is not in the best interests of the client. This is, of course, assuming that other referral sources are possible. Nonetheless, the therapist is not duty bound to continue forever with a noncompliant client, and could well incur legal risk by doing so.

I belong to a professional association that repeatedly publishes statements urging members to provide pro bono or free services. I am open to occasionally helping someone who cannot afford to pay for treatment, but I do not like the idea of being told by a professional association that I have to provide free services. It is easy for the association to say that, but they do not have to pay the bills, I do. If I refuse to give away my services, do I risk being unethical?

It is easy for a professional association to set forth ethical notions, such as pro bono services, because they undergird the association's claim to be in existence to further good for society—which is true. In the realm of ethics, the thrust is aspirational, not mandatory. A law can mandate, but in the particular case of (hypothetically) mandating a professional to provide free services, there would be a plethora of reasons, including Constitutional protections from unlawful taking by the government, that would allow a legal challenge. Therefore, it is certainly honorable to aspire to benefit society, but there has to be a limit on free service.

The viewpoint in the question ("open to occasionally helping someone who cannot afford to pay for treatment") is consonant with the true meaning of pro bono service. Any source, regardless of distinction, that tries to mandate more is suspect and open to challenge.

There are times when the practitioner must be prepared to assert his or her personal rights. For example, if a professional association alleged that it was unethical to not give a specified quantum of pro bono services and the practitioner thinks otherwise, professional responsibility and personal rights justify opposition through whatever channels are reasonable and appropriate.

If a client fails to pay an overdue account, am I correct that privileged communication keeps me from turning the debt over to a collection agency?

Privileged communication precludes releasing certain information (e.g., of a clinical nature) to another source (e.g., a collection agency). It does not, however, preclude providing certain information for reasonable attempts to collect an overdue debt via a collection agency. It is prudent to screen the collection agency to be sure that the tactics used will be lawful and appropriate under the circumstances.

Further, there seems to be a positive correlation between the amount of the debt and the client's readiness to file an ethical, regulatory, or legal complaint against a therapist whenever an effort is made to collect the debt. Stated bluntly, while a debt to a therapist is subject to a collection effort, there is a strong likelihood of retaliation by the client to avoid the collection.

The prudent approach is to have a clear-cut system for payments, agreed to by the client at the onset of treatment and maintained consistently throughout the treatment relationship. This agreement should include the consequence that will be triggered by failure to make payments accordingly. Thus, whenever a deficit accrues outside the established financial perimeter, the agreed upon consequential act, such as termination and referral elsewhere, should be implemented.

It is usually better to terminate a noncompliant client who breaches the service agreement than to continue on with the (foolish?) hope of financial recovery, while all the time there is an evaluation of the risk that the client will take retaliatory legal action against the therapist when collection effort is eventually made. Stated bluntly, it is a disservice to the client and legally foolish for the therapist to allow a deficit in payment for treatment to occur.

Is it unethical to sue a client?

No, it is not unethical per se to sue a client. However, the answer to the preceding question applies in full, assuming that the cause of action against the client is for a financial debt. That is, if the therapist sues the client for an unpaid debt, only certain information can be released to the court proceedings, and the probability increases that the client will file a countersuit against the therapist.

If the cause of action involves other matters, the therapist is no different from any other plaintiff. For example, a client who physically assaults or harasses a therapist is potentially liable, both criminally and civilly.

Therapists need to protect their personal rights. Because they serve clients with mental problems does not eliminate any personal right. All too often, a therapist erroneously believes that the privileged nature of the communications that occurred within the professional services relationship precludes legal action against the client.

8

Framing a Clinical Practice

Professional training programs have generally tended to omit or minimize knowledge and skills that would help the professional to tailor his or her mental health practice to the realities of the marketplace. Rather, the training emphasis is commonly on idealistic notions and practices. Actual practice seldom, if ever, thrives on idealism alone. A successful practice (e.g., financially viable and legally safe) is likely being titrated with a healthy dose of pragmatism.

Creating an effective framework for a mental health practice involves an accurate assessment of one's knowledge and skills. For some practitioners, this is an onerous task. They reason, incorrectly, that to admit to limitations is synonymous with admitting to incompetence or diminished professionalism. On the contrary, it is highly professional to render only those services in which one is competent. This promotes the best interests of the client and society and, at the same time, is sound risk management for the practitioner.

Consideration of market potential is a relevant, but not a controlling, factor in framing a clinical practice. More often than not, exaggerating the need to be highly, as opposed to reasonably,

113

competitive by offering an extensive range of services can lead to poor quality and economic and legal problems.

This chapter attempts to fill the prescriptions for a healthy dose of pragmatism. It recognizes the need to be reasonably competitive, but it also emphasizes that the practitioner should frame the practice on the basis of his or her unique combination of strengths. The discussion also includes legal considerations.

It is my impression that it pays to offer a broad range of services, as opposed to being limited to a few services. Assuming that I could generate an adequate number of clients with either approach, which would be best from a legal perspective?

The fundamental of all legally safe and ethically correct professional practice is competency. The broader the scope of services, the greater the requirement that competency be diversified. Obviously there may be unequal degrees of competency in the different types of services, which ushers in the problem of how to be sure that competency, regardless of type of service, is consonant with the standard of care.

If personal resources (e.g., time, energy, commitment, and money for training) allow, it is feasible to create and maintain competency in a variety of services. On the other hand, it seems self-evident that consolidating those resources to cultivate impeccable competency can offer benefits to both the client and the therapist.

If there is no shortage of clients, it would seem that optimum professionalism would be gained by superior competency in a limited number of areas. If a broad array of services would mean vulnerability to unanticipated or unintended incompetence, a restricted scope of practice would be preferred.

To minimize legal liability, risk taking vis-à-vis practice skills must be avoided. Stated differently, competency to meet the needs of the client according to the applicable professional standard should never be in doubt.

I would like to be recognized as a specialist in a particular kind of service, but I have heard that there may be more legal risk. Is that true?

Receiving treatment from a "specialist" has a certain appeal to the client because it connotes that greater skill and benefits will be embraced. This expectation is recognized by the law when it comes to deciding what standard of care should be applied to alleged malpractice. Commonly, if the client has a reasonable basis for believing that the therapist is a specialist, derived, for example, from how the therapist frames or defines his or her practice, the standard of care required legally will be elevated above what would be required of the nonspecialist or general practitioner.

Yes, by legal principle, being a specialist portends to carry greater risk than being a generalist. To the contrary, if the therapist is, in fact, a specialist, it might be assumed that the specialist has more refined expertise, which ends up lessening the risk of breaching the standard of care. Further, being a specialist has a certain market value; that is, being recognized as being able to provide outstanding professional services will bring clients to the practice. Thus, "to be or not to be" is a question that can only be answered by the therapist according to personal assessment and values. (See page 7 for additional comments on this matter.)

To make sure that I have plenty of clients, I am inclined to accept almost anyone who will come in for an initial session. After a session or two, I may decide to refer them to someone else. I admit, however, that if they can afford my services, I am apt to keep serving them. Does this seem like a reasonable way of operating?

This question reaches, like others, to the matter of competency. Attempting to provide services to everyone seems unwise, since it would require consistent and broad skills. No therapist is properly suited for every would-be client.

Because the client can afford to pay the fee is an appropriate factor to consider before initiating treatment, but it should not be the only or primary factor. Rather, the most important issue is whether or not the therapist can adequately meet the treatment needs of the clients.

In many instances, the issue should extend to consideration of whether or not the therapist can, of the options available, best meet the needs of the client. In other words, part of professional-ism is accepting that the foremost concern is the best interest of the client. It is probable that a certain percentage of clients making an initial contact about treatment would be better served by another source.

While the client's welfare is paramount, the therapist can take solace from recognizing that by being selective, taking only those clients to whom he or she can assuredly provide quality services, there is an endowment of risk management. That is, by weeding out clients with whom it is doubtful that excellence will be achieved or who present an incompatible composite (be it by personality, motivation, or finances), the therapist will benefit and have the best possible clientele from the legal, professional, and business vantage points.

Recommended Readings

In order to maintain a practice-oriented style, the material in this book purposely did not include citations. Without exception, however, every answer is based on a legal and behavioral science authority, as well as what I have experienced firsthand as an attorney protecting mental health practitioners.

For the reader lacking familiarity with the law, I would suggest:

Meyer, R. G., Landis, E. R., & Hays, J. R. (1988). *Law for the psychotherapist*. New York: W. W. Norton.

Also, a book that I wrote with associates covers the broad range of legal fundamentals and applications in mental health; it is:

Woody, R. H. (and Associates) (1984). *The law and practice of human services*. San Francisco: Jossey-Bass.

Readily apparent from the questions and answers, liability is the underlying dimension for the legal aspects of mental health practice. Relatedly, malpractice and standard of care are critical concepts. Perhaps the most scholarly source on these issues, although it covers many other legal matters that lack direct relevance to mental health practice, is:

Keeton, W. P., Dobbs, D. B., Keeton, R. E., & Owen, D. G. (1984). *Prosser and Keeton on torts* (5th ed.). St. Paul, MN: West.

More basic definitions and discussions for mental health practitioners are presented, along with specific suggestions for avoiding malpractice, in my book:

Woody, R. H. (1988). *Fifty ways to avoid malpractice: A guidebook for the mental health practitioner.* Sarasota, FL: Professional Resource Exchange.

As is evident in many of the questions and answers, risk management and business principles must be effectively interfaced with professional notions about mental health practice. I have prepared a three-book series that moves through the essentials for succeeding in practice; those books are:

Woody, R. H. (1988). *Protecting your mental health practice: How to minimize legal and financial risk.* San Francisco: Jossey-Bass.

Woody, R. H. (1989). *Business success in mental health practice: Modern marketing, management and legal strategies.* San Francisco: Jossey-Bass.

Woody, R. H. (1991). *Quality care in mental health services: Assuring the best clinical services.* San Francisco: Jossey-Bass.

For those who provide professional services to children, a useful book is:

Nurcombe, B., & Partlett, D. F. (1994). *Child mental health and the law.* New York: The Free Press (Macmillan).

For an understanding of psychological assessment and providing expert testimony, I would suggest, respectively:

Shapiro, D. L. (1991). *Forensic psychological assessment.* Needham Heights, MA: Allyn and Bacon; and Brodsky, S. L. (1991). *Testifying in court: Guidelines and maxims for the expert witness.* Washington, DC: American Psychological Association.

The difficult decision of fulfilling the duty to warn of dangerousness to self and others is clarified and summarized in:

VandeCreek, L., & Knapp, S. (1993). *Tarasoff and beyond: Legal and clinical considerations in the treatment of life-endangering patients* (rev. ed.). Sarasota, FL: Professional Resource Press.

As a caveat, it is understatement to assert that the mental health professional must be constantly alert to the legal implications of practice and the evolution of the law. The law is always changing, and each jurisdiction has its unique authority. It is regrettable that university training programs have been slow to fulfill the public policy demand for improved legal and ethical considerations by practitioners. Consequently, each practitioner must studiously seek to advance his or her knowledge, such as through continuing education. The author hopes that this book has contributed to that objective.

About the Author

ROBERT HENLEY WOODY is a Professor of Psychology and Social Work at the University of Nebraska at Omaha, and works as an attorney protecting mental health professionals. He holds a Doctor of Philosophy degree in counseling psychology from Michigan State University, a Doctor of Science degree in health services research and administration from the University of Pittsburgh, and a Juris Doctor degree in law from the Creighton University. He is a member of the Florida, Michigan, and Nebraska Bars, and a Licensed Psychologist in Florida and Michigan. He is a Diplomate in Clinical Psychology, ABPP, and Forensic Psychology, ABFP. He is a Fellow of the American Psychological Association and the American Association for Marriage and Family Therapy. He has authored twenty-five books and over one hundred and fifty articles for professional journals. He conducts seminars nationwide on quality care and avoiding malpractice in mental health services. Since 1984, he has authored a "Psycholegal Notebook" column, which appears in publications from a number of state psychological associations.